Much Par

Vertebral Manipulation –
A Part of Orthodox Medicine

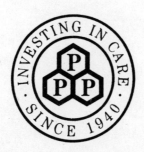

Sincere thanks are due to Private Patients Plan for their generous
sponsorship of this book

True wisdom lies in understanding how little we know
– and acknowledging this

Vertebral Manipulation –
A Part of Orthodox Medicine

John K. Paterson
Les Fitayes, 13640 La Roque D'Anthéron, France

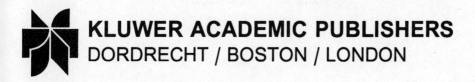

KLUWER ACADEMIC PUBLISHERS
DORDRECHT / BOSTON / LONDON

Coventry University

Distributors

---

for the United States and Canada: Kluwer Academic Publishers, PO Box 358, Accord Station, Hingham, MA 02018-0358, USA
for all other countries: Kluwer Academic Publishers Group, Distribution Center, PO Box 322, 3300 AH Dordrecht, The Netherlands

A catalogue record for this book is available from the British Library.

ISBN 0-7923-8885-2

PO6440

Contents

Appendices

First Foreword

One of the chief demands on health care provision is made by back pain or its derivatives; this is true internationally, whatever system of delivery is employed. In the United Kingdom alone, its cost is many millions of pounds a year. Clinically, there is considerable confusion, as there are numerous schools of thought as to aetiology, diagnosis and therapy in this group of conditions, exhibiting wide differences in both philosophy and practical teaching. Each school's teaching is governed by its particular ideology, not always in accord with proven anatomical and physiological reality, and also by the sociological and political conditions pertaining in the country.

This confusion has had several effects on members of the medical profession. Some have recognized the common, if unpredictable, value of vertebral manipulation, and have accepted 'alternative' teaching somewhat uncritically. At the other extreme, others have rejected it, along with the teaching of a variety of cults, thereby losing a potentially valuable therapy. Many have chosen to ignore the whole subject, but the problem has not 'gone away'! The patient has suffered as a result of this; but a further result is that referral of such cases (particularly to hospitals) runs at an artificially elevated level, significantly boosting the escalating cost of back pain world-wide.

This very unsatisfactory situation is slowly changing. As Chairman of the Scientific Advisory Committee of the International Federation of Manual Medicine, the author of this small book has recently devised and conducted the first international teachers' workshop. In this, he deliberately confronted matters of controversy, subjecting them to critical scrutiny on a scientific basis, and achieving consensus on numerous items. This book reflects the discussions provoked in the workshop, presenting vertebral manipulation as a simple, extremely safe therapy, suitable for wide deployment, particularly in general practice, which has at its core a basis wholly acceptable to the orthodox. It is encouraging that he has been commissioned to conduct a further workshop in 1995.

I welcome this book as a reasoned exposition of an important and difficult problem in health care. Together with the new postgraduate diploma in primary care rheumatology (offered by the University of Bath, in close collaboration with the Primary Care Rheumatology Society), it should make a real contribution to reducing the currently excessive level of expenditure on musculoskeletal problems.

RH McNeilly MSc MD FFCM *January 1995*
Director of Medical Services, Private Patients Plan

Second Foreword

The emphasis in Health Care in many European countries is currently shifting towards primary care led services. Pain of vertebral origin and associated musculo-skeletal disorders are amongst the top three most common presenting problems in general practice, yet the skills and resources for managing them in primary care are often inadequate. In the UK, for example, it is estimated that there are some 14 to 15 million GP consultations anually for back pain alone, presenting a huge challenge in terms of clinical management and cost both to the NHS and private health care. This challenge has been recognized in the UK Government's Health of the Nation Strategy and the recent Report on Back Pain from its Clinical Standards Group. Amongst the recommendations are earlier and more active interventions (including vertebral manipulation), improved primary care management of early back pain and better access to specialist services.

With this book, the author, Dr John Paterson, an experienced GP himself and an authority on musculoskeletal medicine, makes a much needed and timely contribution to the field, particularly in the area of vertebral manipulation. It is published at a time when patients and health care managers are demanding high clinical standards, together with closer scrutiny of the cost–effectiveness of interventions. In answering this challenge, the medical profession must deploy 'evidence-based clinical practice' approaches wherever possible; abandoning outdated behaviours and using only those with proven effectiveness.

The processes of literature search and peer review, the challenging of assumptions, the establishment of common terminology, of standards for clinical record-keeping and consensus on the clinical effectiveness of basic manipulation are the building blocks of evidence-based practice. They are also essential to the development of education programmes so necessary to ensure implementation of clinical guidelines.

The very prevalence of back pain together with evidence that effective early treatments including vertebral manipulation can prevent long-term disability are strong arguments for a revolution in learning and teaching about musculoskeletal medicine. The author is right to suggest that undergraduate and postgraduate training programmes should be revised to include this important area of clinical practice as a priority. More opportunities to learn vertebral manipulation should be available to established GPs as part of well-planned higher professional education, higher degree courses and continuing professional development. Doctors should be trained to work in multidisciplinary teams with other health practitioners in this field and to understand the roles of generalists, specialists, the professions allied to medicine and complementary therapists. All should be prepared to work to agreed standards, to review continually their own performance and overall outcomes.

Such actions, together with publications like this one, will help to establish vertebral manipulation and related techniques as orthodox medical practice – many of them hopefully as routine primary care procedures. Research suggests this could have a major impact in reducing long-term disability for many thousands of patients annually throughout the European Union. In turn the heavy personal and public economic burdens consequent on vertebral and associated disorders could be substantially reduced.

Robert M. Berrington
GP Regional Adviser
Anglia/Oxford Regional Health Authority and University of Cambridge

Introduction

This small book requires some explanation. It has long been recognized that the chief importance of managing the whole complex of pain of vertebral origin lies in the extremely common incidence of its constituent components, rather than in the intrinsic features any of its number may present. Back pain may at first seem a dull and unimportant subject, so diminishing the significance of vertebral manipulation, but, as will be discussed in this book, pain of vertebral origin presents in a wide range of guises. Largely due to the twin phenomena of referred pain and referred tenderness, these are far more numerous than the simple back ache which may at first be imagined. They include head pain, brachial pain, thoracic and abdominal pain, as well as the well-recognized sciatica[1-4].

Because of their very common incidence, substantial improvements of their management within the medical profession would clearly be of advantage to the patient, but this is possible only on two conditions being satisfied:

1. Assessment of the whole range of musculoskeletal problems must be based as far as possible on accurately measured observation, rather than on unsubstantiated beliefs.

2. It must be clearly shown how reappraisal of these very common problems may indicate logical changes in therapeutic approach.

At present the medical profession is deeply divided as to what role (if any) vertebral manipulation should play in the management of a number of musculoskeletal conditions, but, before making any meaningful assessment of this, the current very unsatisfactory situation in this field has to be reviewed in some detail.

Vertebral manipulation has been practised for thousands of years all over the world. Hippocrates taught it. At some stage the medical profession abandoned it as a part of orthodoxy possibly for fear of contagion, certainly not as a result of proof of inefficacy or danger, although this is still canvassed by some and widely believed. In the United Kingdom, it continued to be offered by the bone-setters, which remains the case today. For up to one hundred and twenty years, under one name or another, numerous more or less sophisticated versions of vertebral manipulation have been taught. Their names are many, their ideological precepts astonishingly varied; they do not need to be detailed here, though some of their theoretical bases need to be evaluated. A selection of the major controversial items is discussed in Part II.

However, in spite of these teachings being vigorously promoted, both politically and right across the media, and although their several faces have been widely, it erratically, accepted by the public, in few countries has vertebral manipulation regained the whole-hearted support of the orthodox medical profession. Has this been due to 'pig-headedness' on the part of too conservative and protectionist a medical profession? Does it reveal a solid scepticism, born of a belief in scientific principles not always found to be wholly adopted by other disciplines (nor, for that matter, consistently within its own ranks)? Or is there any other reason for the current rather unsatisfactory situation?

These were the questions which, in 1993, prompted the Fédération Internationale de Médecine Manuelle (FIMM) to promote an international workshop for teachers in this field, with the object of establishing guidelines for teaching musculoskeletal medicine in member countries, as a part of orthodox medicine. The proposition was first made a year before by Joan Garcia-Alsina, Professor of Rehabilitation in Barcelona, and it was further contained in a paper I presented at the same meeting[5]. The resultant workshop, held in Vienna in 1994, proved a fascinating venture, having at its core a handbook, *An Acceptable Face to Musculoskeletal Medicine*[6], upon which this book is substantially modelled.

It is widely known that numerous 'schools' of vertebral manipulation exist, both within the medical profession and without, and it is also well appreciated that the teaching of these individual schools has differed considerably in the past, and still does; differed, that is, both from orthodox teaching, and also one school from another. This is strikingly illustrated in the book of the 1989 Congress of FIMM, *Back Pain – An International Review*[7]. Here are to be found many conflicting views, from the serious scientific studies which make up the bulk of Part I to those expressed in parts II and III: many were presented as the truth, some of which seem to reflect fantasy in preference to fact, at times choosing to ignore evidence not well suited to preconceived ideas. While some may feel it to be so, this statement is not over-critical; it is one of all-too-well-validated fact. The problem is seen to be both widespread and international.

The effect of the spate of material of varying validity upon the orthodox medical profession over a very substantial period has taken three major forms. At one extreme, vertebral manipulation has been embraced by a few doctors as being wholly legitimate, together with the accompanying ideology preached by the particular cult concerned. This is, of course, a relatively 'easy option', in that, without undue heartache, it allows the doctor to treat a substantial number of patients with a reasonable expectation of success and in the comforting belief that he knows what he is doing. This is a trend which is increasing quite rapidly, but it has obvious dangers and some items of faith have been shown to be erroneous.

Midway, it has long been regarded by a substantial proportion of doctors as a hopefully harmless eccentricity in its proponents. This stance, while it is in no way damaging to the practice of vertebral manipulation, is a somewhat negative attitude.

At the other extreme, it has been discarded by many, along with its flawed rationale. (It is discouraging that, even in 1994, anyone should have represented vertebral manipulation as being highly dangerous, without a shred of evidence to back the claim other than a solitary instance of delayed diagnosis[8].) It is clear that none of these three attributes is really sound; nor do either the second or third of them contribute positively to the well-being of the patient.

However, there is a further factor which does seem to have been at play in some countries at least; the personalities of some of the proponents of vertebral manipulation. In some instances, this appears to have contributed to rejection of this therapy simply because the more orthodox have felt they were being 'steam-rollered' by somewhat opinionated heretics. Their predictable response has been to retreat into the security of the 'establishment', in the face of what they saw as an assault, firmly closing the door both on these individuals and on the therapies they practised and preached.

None-the-less, it certainly seems that it is in substantial part because of the wide disparity of teaching that the orthodox medical profession has to date on the whole remained somewhat aloof – and who could blame them? In view of their demonstrable differences, and despite their often deeply ingrained certitudes, the various protagonists of what may be lumped together as musculoskeletal medicine cannot all be right! It we are not to dismiss them out of hand, can their various claims be measured against some sort of standard? If so, which standard is to be utilized? Is there not, running through the vertebral moiety of musculoskeletal medicine, an identifiable scientific core acceptable to the orthodox; if there is, what does it look like? If we are to identify such a core, a very basic non-controversial approach is clearly indicated; non-controversial from an orthodox viewpoint.

This is what this small book seeks to provide, and, at once, it becomes apparent that I am addressing myself to two separate groups of doctors: to those whose enthusiasm may perhaps in the past have overridden their self-criticism, as well as to those whose very natural reactive scepticism possibly clouds their ability to view the subject wholly objectively (a situation in some instances fostered by the personalities involved). To achieve this, it is first necessary to consider precisely what the orthodox medical profession legitimately requires in order to be persuaded that vertebral manipulation is scientifically acceptable. This is discussed in Chapter 1.

In the light of this approach, critical evaluation of some of the current teaching and literature in this field reveals failure to meet these criteria as being alarmingly common. Indeed, one of the internationally best-known teachers in musculoskeletal medicine has recently declared his agreement that palpation is an immeasurable subjective impression[9], while continuing to use it as his chief diagnostic criterion! I find it difficult to accept what I see as a marriage of two absolute incompatibles. The wider realization of the importance and extent of this sort of intellectual anomaly was one of the chief results of last year's international teachers' workshop in Vienna.

In view of the current wave of public popularity of a number of therapeutic measures, particularly vertebral manipulation, it is profitable to examine critically some of the major hypotheses to be found in current musculoskeletal teaching, be it orthodox, alternative or complementary, so as to make a more objective assessment of their validity vis-à-vis scientifically validated beliefs. Where such ideas are found wanting, they must be identified and either abandoned or presented as no more than hypotheses; *but there may well be no necessity to abandon the therapies they promote if these can be justified scientifically.*

One crucial and positive question needs to be answered.

Can vertebral manipulation be justified on an orthodox medical basis, without recourse to ideologies found to be seriously flawed?

This book seeks to provide an answer to this. The international teachers' workshop certainly demonstrated that it can.

Teachers must be constantly alert to this question; *far from being absolute, scientific truth is necessarily ever transient.* Indeed, the process of learning often demands the abandonment of beliefs previously held – on the adduction of compelling evidence showing them to be erroneous. *Failure to do this simply means failure to learn.* Not only must the orthodox medical profession be prepared to accept some facets of alternative teaching, alternative therapists of any persuasion (medically qualified, or not) must also be prepared to accept scientifically sound evidence, and *must act upon it*, abandoning discredited hypotheses. Many must learn to accept criticism of their current beliefs as a bid for scientific advance, rather than as a personal attack. Those who wish to explore questions of scientific bases and their validation in greater detail are referred to *Musculoskeletal Medicine, the Spine*[10].

To a substantial extent based on that employed (with serial changes) by Burn and myself since 1983, the syllabus outlined in this book has evolved further through discussion in the first international teachers' workshop. Its object is to lay down guidelines for elementary musculoskeletal medicine teaching, aimed at providing the novice with a scientifically sound basis for practice in this field, in safety and with reasonable expectation of therapeutic success. It is to be found in Appendix 4. It does not extend to the more sophisticated diagnostic or therapeutic techniques advocated by many, being deliberately restricted to those few which have been shown to have bases which are scientifically valid. Neither does it cater for the quite different requirements of specialist practice, although, to be acceptable, the latter must, of course, be based on equally sound principles. This last very important matter is explored more fully in Chapter 20.

The necessity for such basic teaching to be supported by texts which are themselves scientifically acceptable cannot be too strongly stressed. Regardless of their origins, orthodox or complementary, all hypotheses must be subjected to the same degree of critical evaluation. Likewise, new and relevant evidence must *always* demand re-examination of current beliefs and teaching. While this may seem obvious, it remains a common finding for much musculoskeletal literature to appear distinctly rigid.

Notable recommended exclusions from the basic syllabus are five in number; all from a diagnostic point of view. They also are given in Appendix 4, together with the reasons for their exclusion, although discussed in greater detail in the appropriate chapters. They are: spinal joint mobility, vertebral position, axial muscle strength testing, clinical biomechanics, and posture and gait. As will be found from the text, these exclusions aroused considerable discussion in the workshop; it is stressed that their exclusion is deliberate, limited to basic teaching, and does not necessarily imply that they have no place in musculoskeletal medicine. Of course, in the event of the adduction of sound evidence in their favour, they may well be returned to a future basic syllabus.

It is sometimes suggested that vertebral manipulation is a difficult art to learn; yet, throughout history, the majority of its (commonly successful) practitioners have had no formal training at all! In view of the currently known physiology, a very basic training is all that is required by the interested doctor, *provided that the contraindications are consistently recognized and rigidly observed*. I am on record as saying that, "if you can ride a bicycle and play a better than average game of ping-pong, you can quickly learn to manipulate the spine". Such a readily acquired competence reflects a level of neuromuscular co-ordination wholly adequate for the employment of the simple physiologically based measures advocated. There can be little scientific justification for the teaching of numerous, sophisticated, complex and subtly differing techniques, based on unvalidated hypotheses.

It may be asked whether whole-hearted acceptance of vertebral manipulation by the orthodox medical profession matters very much. I submit that it matters for four cogent reasons:

1. It is a rapidly deployable, remarkably safe therapeutic option, which may prove useful for a very large number of patients.

2. Its inclusion within orthodoxy will enhance the potential armamentarium of the medical profession; particularly in general practice, where it may further be of financial advantage to the doctor.

3. It is likely to speed up the availability of therapy for an enormous number of patients who currently have to wait too long for any effective treatment.

4. It represents a substantial saving in the cost of health care provision, whatever its mode of funding and delivery.

It is proposed that the wide use of a syllabus for basic teaching, such as appears in Appendix 4, will contribute to the acceptance of musculoskeletal medicine within the orthodox medical profession, internationally. Perhaps the most important factor in its acceptability is that it contains no 'factual' material which is not validated. Details will change with the demands of continuing research, but its basis must remain scientific. A core of a few countries adopting this syllabus will further permit the exchange of teachers and other forms of international co-ordination within the Fédération Internationale Médecine Manuelle. More advanced teaching may readily be grafted onto such an orthodox base, thereby largely avoiding the difficulties inevitably encountered in trying to establish a medical speciality without the benefit of an adequate scientific platform. Most important, the patient will see, in this fresh medical interest in the problem, a gleam of hope for the future management of many of his pains. Finally, not only may those already interested in the field find here some sober explanation of what they are doing, but their strongest critics will at last see scientific justification for some of their enthusiasms.

I am greatly indebted to all those who responded to my several questionnaires, without which I could not have made sound progress, either with the workshop or with this book, but chiefly to Professor Joan Garcia-Alsina for his invaluable help on the education subcommittee of FIMM and for his enthusiastic support of the workshop. Also, I have to thank Professor Hans Tilscher, President of FIMM, for his whole-hearted encouragement from the beginning, and my colleague of many years' standing, Dr Loic Burn, for his constant constructive criticism and for permitting me to make use of material from our previous books. I am also happy to acknowledge the vital role played by all participants in that workshop. (See Appendix 1.)

I am most grateful to Dr R.H. McNeilly (Director of Health Services, Private Patients Plan) for writing a foreword to this book, stressing the social importance of the inclusion of vertebral manipulation within orthodoxy. I also have to thank Dr Robert Berrington (Regional Adviser in General Practice, Anglia/Oxford Regional Health Authority and the University of Cambridge) for writing an additional foreword, underlining the clinical importance of musculoskeletal medicine and the need for the incorporation of vertebral manipulation in general practice. I wish to express my sincere gratitude to Private Patients Plan for their generous sponsorship of the workshop and this book, without which both would have been impossible. Last of all, I have to mention the unfailing help of Dr Peter Clarke and Phil Johnstone, of Kluwer Academic Publishers, both in guiding my erring steps and in performing their parts of the task with all speed.

John K. Paterson   *January 1995*
Chairman, Scientific Advisory Committee, FIMM

PART I

Part I of this small book presents a simple basis upon which vertebral manipulation may be taught and practised in safety, with reasonable expectation of therapeutic success and without recourse to controversial hypotheses. In this way, it is scientifically acceptable to the orthodox medical profession, and it must be stressed that, coupled with a surprisingly brief practical course of instruction in techniques, it is sufficient for the novice to make use of this potentially valuable therapeutic option.

1
Prerequisites for a scientifically acceptable musculoskeletal approach

---

First, it is necessary to consider precisely what the orthodox medical profession legitimately requires in order to be persuaded that vertebral manipulation is scientifically acceptable. Its chief demands are seven:

1. At all times, a clear distinction must be made between proven fact and hypothesis. Any statement presented as fact must be supported by valid evidence. Where the available evidence is seen to be conflicting, this conflict must be aired, rather than swept under the carpet, and a reasoned explanation must be afforded as to why one particular interpretation is preferred to another.

2. Quotations of statements of fact or of hypothesis must be accurate, and they must be clearly categorized as one or the other. Reporting what has not been written and 'selling' hypothesis as truth are both intellectually no less than dishonest, and these are things all must look for, both in the personal teaching and in the supporting texts encountered. There is a parallel to this to be found in certain reviews of books; the reviewer who criticizes what has not been written, either because he fails to read the text with sufficient care, or because he thinks he knows what the author is going to say!

3. Adequate referencing is mandatory; recourse to bald statements, unsupported by independent evidence, smacks of the 'I can tell' syndrome, which must ever remain anathema to the serious doctor and an impediment to scientific progress[11]. Here, it is worth while adding that it is poor practice to refer to work that remains unpublished; after all, the primary objective of giving a reference is to enable the reader to refer to the work quoted!

4. In original work, several standards need to be met. Sample size must be adequate for the subject under review. While rare conditions are necessarily studied in small numbers, it is *quite unacceptable* to draw conclusions from a study of a small sample in conditions of common occurrence. The population from which the sample is drawn must be clearly identified. Data must be objectively measurable, to a known degree of accuracy; while subject report is to be avoided wherever possible. Only when the foregoing standards are met, may analysis be made; and then either it must be made in statistically acceptable form, or the result must be presented from the outset as being

8

statistically insignificant. (In the latter case, the work may still be publishable, as a useful and interesting commentary, or as a stimulus to further research, although it will, of course, carry less weight than work which is statistically significant.)

5. Clarity of reporting is fundamental; at times it may be obscured by the imperfections of translation between languages. Where the latter is needed, it is often wise to have a draft checked by a native speaker of the language of presentation. Such a person should be chosen with care!

6. Jargon must be avoided as far as possible, other than that which is common to the medical profession in general; inevitably its wider use labels the writer as a believer in a particular set of values; values which may be found questionable when subjected to independent scrutiny.

7. Illustration needs to show something as clearly and as simply as possible; too much information in a single illustration serves only to confuse the reader. It is better by far to make use of several illustrations. Radiographs and various scans are sometimes difficult to reproduce in print without loss of clarity; photographs are a poor medium for illustrating diagnostic or therapeutic manoeuvres; line drawings should be as simple as possible, the use of several colours sometimes making the illustration clearer (though more expensive to produce); linear graphs and bar graphs are well suited to reproduction and are sufficient for most statistical purposes. Some more bizarre forms of illustration confuse the reader still further and should be avoided. *If any form of illustration does not clarify the text, it is better omitted.* Further, the matter illustrated must be as near the truth as possible, in turn supported by the best evidence available.

Ideally, clinical teaching of vertebral manipulation should be supported by texts which meet *all* the requirements set out above. While this may be a counsel of perfection, it is certainly necessary to be very selective in choosing texts for teaching, if they are to prove widely acceptable. Teaching must further stress the serious limitations of subjective impressions, such as the palpatory assessment of bony position, tissue texture and joint movement. There are four limitations:

1. They are individual to each observer.
2. They are effectively immeasurable in a clinical setting.
3. They are thereby non-repeatable in a scientific sense.
4. They are therefore ill-suited to statistical analysis.

Their use is thus an example of faith rather than of fact; they cannot be scientifically acceptable.

Work which satisfies these requirements demands acceptance by the orthodox medical profession, provided it demonstrates benefit to the patient.

2
Epidemiology of back pain

Why consider this subject at all? Some countries ignore it in musculoskeletal teaching, contributing to the wide discrepancies found between nations[5]. (See also Appendix 2.) I believe that, currently, undergraduate teaching of the subject is commonly inadequate for our purpose, and that its exclusion from basic courses in musculoskeletal medicine detracts from the authenticity of such teaching, thus reducing the chance of musculoskeletal medicine being accepted by orthodoxy in those countries which omit it. An appreciation of the potential sources and causes of back pain is an essential part of any serious medical approach, suggesting possible avenues of therapeutic and prophylactic management, as also of research.

Moreover, there are three widely held beliefs which are damaging to general acceptance; that the incidence of back pain is related to: skeletal defect, to degenerative changes and ageing, and to a variety of postural deformities. Contrary to such beliefs, the truth, as shown below, is otherwise.

1. There is NO proven correlation between back pain and skeletal defect[12].
2. There is NO proven correlation between back pain and degenerative changes[13], except when those changes are gross.
3. There is NO proven correlation between back pain and postural deformity[14], unless this is gross.

There are four major difficulties in assessing back pain data.

1. Definitions of pain are numerous, thus at times rendering comparison invalid[15].

2. Much depends upon patient report; well known to be unreliable[16]. The use of visual analogue scales is often misleading, as a high proportion of patients indicate the middle third of the range as being appropriate to their condition[16].

3. Factors which may influence the incidence of back pain are multiple and often co-existent[17].

4. In part as a result of these factors, diagnosis is seldom valid, making research the more difficult[10]. This unwelcome fact is underlined by the plethora of syndromes to be found, all idiosyncratic descriptions of what *may be*!

No-one disputes that the epidemiological scale of the problem is enormous

10

internationally. The figures vary widely, according to their source and the criteria employed in their collection; they are thus not truly comparable. However, all agree that they are very big. The cost of the problem is in keeping with its size; to the patient, to the insurance agencies, to the state health care systems, to industry and, indirectly, to the individual national economies. However, sickness rates are unreliable, due to the difficulty already mentioned – including the common invalidity of diagnosis. Certification is thereby often misleading, with the result that the relevant statistics are necessarily suspect.

There is *some* not wholly satisfactory evidence of a causal relationship between back pain and physically heavy work, static work postures, frequent bending and twisting, lifting and other forceful movements, repetitive work and vibration[18-20]. This statement goes as far as is scientifically legitimate – some relationship! It remains too vague for more specific representation.

There is again some relationship between back pain and genetic factors, such as HLA-B27[21]. An evolutionary cause is not supported by the currently available evidence[22]. Age, gender and posture are poorly correlated with back pain, the latter including differences in leg length, popularly thought to be of significance[23,24]. Neither is there a convincing case made for the association of physical fitness with a reduction in incidence, severity or duration of episodes of back pain, again due to the impossibility of isolating individual factors in a clinical setting[25].

Ergonomic studies to date have proved inconclusive[26]. Radiology and various other scanning techniques are reviewed in Chapter 12.

Only two sound conclusions may be drawn from these considerations.

1. We have a big complex problem, in which many factors are involved, usually inseparable from each other, and thereby individually immeasurable.

2. In part as a result of this, management of pain of vertebral origin commonly remains empirical: this demands change of therapy at an early stage, when improvement is found to be lacking or unacceptably slow.

A clear understanding of these two conclusions, both within musculoskeletal medicine and amongst the more sceptical of the orthodox, is a vital prerequisite to the acceptance of musculoskeletal medicine by orthodoxy. Claims to the contrary are, without exception, damaging to the chances of such acceptance. The 'I can tell' syndrome is seen to be potentially very harmful. Omission of the whole subject of epidemiology from basic teaching is similarly unacceptable to the orthodox. We certainly need a basic understanding of the epidemiology of pain of vertebral origin, even if our knowledge is necessarily limited; and we need to be clear about those limitations. It is interesting to note that, of the five participants in the workshop who reported the current exclusion of the subject from their natural teaching, three accepted its importance by the end, hoping to alter their respective national syllabi on return.

3
Pain perception and modulation

The complexity of pain perception is enormous. It is also now very much better understood than was the case a number of years ago. As in any scientific endeavour, new evidence, properly processed, leads to new knowledge, which must show some beliefs to be no longer tenable. It must be unscientific to cling to beliefs which have been shown to be erroneous.

Modern technology has permitted a more detailed understanding of (in particular) nociception and mechanoception, and much is now known about the chemistry of pain[27]. The anatomy of nociceptive and mechanoceptive nerve endings is well documented, as are their distribution and behaviour, as well as the related afferent terminations[28]. (An exception to this statement is found in respect of the annulus fibrosus, where argument still rages with regard to innervation; this argument is purely academic, as the annulus is so closely applied to the anterior and posterior longitudinal ligaments, which are well supplied. Anything distorting the one must distort the other.)

The gate theory is very soundly established, and this is fundamental to several musculoskeletal therapies[29]. The dorsal horn is the site of much relevant activity, mapped in its laminae in great detail[30].

Transmission pathways are seen to be important, and endogenous pain control mechanisms play a vital part, via endorphin-mediated analgesia systems (EMAS), the peri-aqueductal grey (PAG), and the rostral ventro-medial (RVM) medulla[31]. Most important, there is seen to be a profound difference between the mechanism of acute pain and that of chronic pain[32]. A more detailed overview of these matters is to be found in *Musculoskeletal Medicine, the Spine*[10]. What matters here is that we appreciate the clinical significance of this broadened understanding. The only *certain* mechanism whereby manipulation works remains inhibition of C-fibres by A-fibre activity.

The wide ramification of nerve fibres up and down the neuraxis (as well as outside the spinal column altogether) is of the greatest significance, as is the realization that, largely because of this, the so-called facilitated cord segment can exist only in the imagination[10]! And, of course, the same applies to the concept of autonomic pain as a separate entity[10]. These remain dreams, and, as such, should be discarded from our teaching.

The significance of this enhanced understanding to the musculoskeletal medicine practitioner could not be greater:

1. The complexity and unpredictability of the relevant structures and activities are paramount.

2. This precludes any possibility of predicting either the incidence of pain, its severity, or the constantly changing realities of muscle function.

3. It further demonstrates, beyond any doubt at all, that the clinician normally remains an empiricist, whether he likes it or not!

4. Any system, diagnostic or therapeutic, which relies on even a minor degree of supposed predictability in this sphere must be viewed with caution. The reality is different.

In practice, this is all the clinician needs to know about how vertebral manipulation works; it works by the inhibition of C-fibres, as a result of stimulation of A-fibres, and best results may be expected where this fact has been exploited to the full. A shrewd awareness of the essentials, of their limitations and of their significance is more important to the patient than a battery of hypotheses. Subject to the rigid observation of the contraindications to manipulation (see Chapter 8), our aim must be to provoke maximum A-fibre activity by judicious exploitation of the known physiology.

4
Referred pain and tenderness

As will become apparent, in the common absence of a valid diagnosis, these twin phenomena are fundamental to scientifically acceptable musculoskeletal case analysis.

The complexity of innervation of the spine, "accounts for the accepted difficulty of determining the anatomical source of low back pain in patients"[33]. Three facts are fundamental to an understanding of referred pain and tenderness: one anatomical, one physiological, one pathological.

1. Nociceptive afferents from visceral tissues project onto the same cells in lamina 5 of the basal spinal nucleus as do the afferents from segmentally related areas of skin[33].

2. Because of this convergence of visceral and cutaneous nociceptive inputs on the relaying cells of lamina 5, their excitation is the essential prerequisite for centripetal transmission of nociceptive activity into the brain, and thus the evocation of the experience of pain[33].

3. It will be apparent that normally trivial stimuli applied to related areas of skin may induce these relay cells to fire, should their excitability be sufficiently increased by pre-existing afferent activity emanating from visceral nociceptive nerve endings[33].

It follows that the original concept of the dermatome as a fixed entity is erroneous: indeed, it has been shown to vary enormously in extent[34]. Further, the same cells in lamina 6 of the dorsal horn have a multiplicity of functions, subserving different functions at different times, their receptive fields varying from a fraction of a dermatome to a whole leg[35]. Therefore, use of the dermatome as more than a topographical marker is unphysiological, and thereby wholly unacceptable.

Tenderness is pain provoked by a normally innocuous stimulus. Tenderness may be referred in exactly the same way as may pain from other causes. Trigger points and tender points would appear to be manifestations of referred pain and tenderness.

Clearly, the use of localization of pain or tenderness as a diagnostic criterion in defining the syndrome is unsound. The reality is that the same pattern of pain and tenderness may arise in different structures at different times in the same individual, as well as in different individuals. The syndrome is thus at all times suspect[10].

14

Nonetheless, these twin phenomena may be put to good use in musculo-skeletal medicine. Together with reflex muscle guarding (wholly acceptable to the orthodox, and an indispensable part of local examination of the back), they form the basis of the skin rolling test and the demonstration of trigger points, alerting the clinician to a range of related possible sources[36]. (See Chapters 10 and 11.) With its extension to deeper structures (e.g. joint capsules), localized tenderness is an accurate indicator for the appropriate delivery site of numerous therapies.

It is the summation of the local physical signs which affords the clinician a sound indication as to the segmental level of origin of pain; not only is this commonly the best he can achieve (with the possible addition of the side affected) but, with a clear understanding and observance of the indications and contraindications for manipulation, it is often all that is necessary for making therapeutic decisions.

Discussion of this matter in the workshop was interesting, most participants finding difficulty in being 'deprived' of a diagnosis, although appreciating the difficulties in making a valid one. It is to be hoped that it will prove possible to rationalize this problem in the second workshop, due to be held in 1995.

Better no diagnosis than one which is invalid!

5
The psychology of pain

This subject is important to musculoskeletal medicine in two major respects.

1. In understanding the psychological components of pain, their inseparability from the somatic components and the difficulties of their clinical assessment (both acute and chronic).

2. In relation to the possible employment of psychological therapies (in chronic intractable pain).

It is important to remember that pain is inevitably the patient's individual, current, transient, emotional response to injury; it is both sensory and cognitive in nature, whatever other elements may be superadded. *Pain is essentially a psychosomatic phenomenon.* Those who choose to use the term psychosomatic in a dismissive or derogatory way display an unfortunate ignorance of the nature of pain. Our more critical colleagues might feel tempted to the view that those who use the term in this way are not best suited to deal with the symptom of pain.

Has pain a function? Acute pain, starting with phasic pain, is commonly thought of as a warning sign, to permit or provoke evasive action or prophylactic inaction[37]. It does not persist beyond the period of healing of the related injury.

On the other hand, chronic pain starts some time after injury (of whatever nature) so it is generally ineffective as a warning. It persists beyond the healing time of related tissue damage[37]. But its chronicity has far-reaching effects in the sufferer, physically, psychologically and socially. These long-term effects include fear, irritability, somatic preoccupation, erratic search for relief of pain and depression[38]. These in turn have their effects on others, thereby adding a social dimension to chronic pain, including that in relation to health care professionals[39]. The chronic pain patient is thereby the more difficult to deal with.

Anxiety is a common and potent cause of both increase in reported severity and attenuation of pain[40]. Psychotic hallucination is a rare cause[41]. At all times it is necessary to consider the patient as a whole, which demands paying attention to psychological, social and environmental factors, as well as demonstrating physical ones. However, differentiation between pain of organic and non-organic origin is often difficult. Numerous attempts have been made to do this, such as the MPPI and the McGill questionnaire[42,43]. But it must be remembered that failure to distinguish an organic cause for pain may sometimes be due to failure to look for the appropriate local physical signs[36]. In this way, abnormal illness behaviour may be erroneously identified. This is, of course, of fundamental importance in musculoskeletal medicine.

Numerous attempts have been made to measure abnormal illness behaviour, none with wholly satisfactory results. From a more practical clinical point of view, pain may be regarded as having four components.

1. Nociception, which has been discussed in Chapter 3.

2. Sensation, which derives from the immensely complex processing of those signals which from time to time traverse the gate.

3. Suffering, which depends upon so many other factors as to form an unsatisfactory index of disability.

4. Altered behaviour. This is relatively easily observed and to some extent measurable.

It must be constantly borne in mind that there is NO positive correlation between the degree of noxious stimulus and the intensity of pain stemming from it[44].

In spite of these difficulties in musculoskeletal medicine, some sort of clinical assessment of pain is of great importance, in particular with a view to making sound therapeutic decisions. This applies both initially and (because therapy is fundamentally empirical in this field) in monitoring alterations of the level of pain essential to further decisions regarding change of therapy. Placebo effect has to be mentioned; it is a proven phenomenon, occurring to a very much greater extent in clinical practice than in laboratory experiments. It is not only commonly of value to the patient (whether he is aware of it or not, and whether he likes it or not) but it demands positive exploitation by the clinician. Those who decry placebo effect fail to appreciate the potential value of a most useful therapeutic option.

What of the clinical parameters of pain?

1. Subject report is known to be pretty unreliable; so it should be avoided as far as possible. For this reason, it also commands minimum significance in case analysis.

2. Behavioural assessment is more objective and to some extent measurable; thereby it is the more reliable. For this reason, it should be given far greater significance in case analysis.

3. Physiological assessment remains objective: it is of greater value for this reason. Scientifically acceptable case analysis must rely as far as possible on measurable indices: referred tenderness and reflex guarding offer an opportunity not to be neglected. It is difficult to 'fudge' these issues!

17

Where pain has become chronic and intractable, psychological therapeutic measures may be of great help[10]. These encompass biofeedback, hypnosis, relaxation techniques (including the Alexander technique), behavioural therapy and cognitive behavioural therapy. Awareness of these therapies is important for ensuring appropriate referral of such patients to pain clinics or directly to a variety of experts. But it is not reasonable to include them in a basic syllabus. Psychological pain is dealt with more fully in *Musculoskeletal Medicine, the Spine*[10].

6
Relevant anatomy

This chapter is not intended to present the subject in its entirety; it is rather offered as a guide to those aspects of anatomy which are of particular importance to the would-be vertebral manipulator.

General

The general conformation of the spinal column is of a series of vertebrae, strung together in such a way as to provide a relatively stable structure which none-the-less permits limited movement at all levels, varying in degree from region to region. The physical variations in bony form are wide, as demanded by the differing functions at successive levels. The manner of connection varies, the basic pattern being that of a single anterior joint (two adjacent vertebrae being separated by an intervertebral disc) and paired posterior joints, which are synovial in type. All three joints are in different planes.

At once, it is obvious that no spinal joint can ever move in isolation, and that the intervertebral joint and its posterior joints must always move in different ways. In practice, of course, neither does any mobile segment ever move in relation to a single neighbour, large regions of the spine inevitably moving at the same time, physiologically, diagnostically or therapeutically (see Chapter 16).

The intervertebral disc is considered in Chapter 17. Here, it is necessary first to remind the reader of its essential structure: the laminated, fibro-elastic annulus fibrosus (very firmly attached above and below), the readily deformable nucleus pulposus and the cartilaginous plates; and that its supporting ligaments are weakest posteriorly. Interminable arguments regarding the innervation of the annulus fibrosus are fruitless for the clinician, as it is well known that the posterior ligament (intimately adherent to the annulus) is richly supplied, and one cannot be damaged without the other.

It is worth while remembering that the articular processes and the posterior vertebral joints are normally asymmetrical, as are the spinous processes and the transverse processes. The posterior joints are synovial in construction, thereby being subject to the degenerative changes common to all synovial joints. Being deep to many structures, palpatory assessment of position must remain wholly hypothetical (see Chapter 14).

The comprehensive arrangement of ligaments is well known: obviously they are stronger in regions of greater strain. They include the following:

1. The anterior longitudinal ligament.
2. The posterior longitudinal ligament.
3. The ligamentum flavum – least well supplied with nociceptors.
4. The ileolumbar ligament.
5. The intertransverse ligaments.
6. The interspinous ligaments.
7. The supraspinous ligaments.
8. Those supporting the capsules of the posterior joints.

The important variations in pattern are dealt with below.

Muscle function (and the testing of individual muscle strength) are dealt with in Chapter 15. Suffice it to say here that the realities are not always what might be expected!

The segmental nerve supply is well known. It is worth reminding the reader that this is commonly subject to overlap to a considerable degree, both within the spinal cord and without; indeed, the posterior rami of L1 and L2 have been shown to supply the upper buttock[45].

It should be remembered that the spinal cord ends about the level of the first lumbar vertebral body; again, this is subject to some variation, but it remains important to the clinician contemplating epidural injection.

It should also be remembered that spinal stenosis may be present (as described by Porter[46]).

Anomalies are common. Lumbo-sacral asymmetry is common – often asymptomatic. The cervico-thoracic junction, the thoraco-lumbar junction and the lumbo-sacral junction have been described as being 'ontogenetically restless' areas. In this connection, the lumbo-sacral angle is intimately connected with differences in leg length and is thereby possibly of importance in posture[24].

Regional

The odontoid process of the atlas is important, as discussed in Chapter 8, as it is a potential site of rheumatoid arthritis. The alar ligaments and the transverse ligament of the axis are important for the same reason, there being no more than 7 mm 'play' between the internal AP diameter of the spinal canal and that of the spinal cord at this level.

The vertebral artery is important as its course is tortuous between C2 and the foramen magnum, swinging laterally through the foramina of the transverse processes of the atlas, and medially again to enter the skull. In this course, it is liable to become kinked, with possibly disastrous effect on the blood supply to the circle of Willis.

Cervical ribs are a potential problem but may be of no consequence. The thoracic spinous processes may mislead the clinician by their obliquity, their tips being approximately at a level with the bodies of the vertebrae caudal to them.

They may also cause confusion by their common asymmetry, suggesting a vertebral rotation where none is present.

Apart from being relatively sturdy, there is little noteworthy about the lumbar vertebrae. The pelvic joints are considered in Chapter 18.

7
Relevant pathology

A clear understanding of this subject is fundamental to safe vertebral manipulation, underpinning the contraindications. At the same time, it should be remembered that significant pathological changes occur relatively rarely, in contradistinction to the commonly reversible mechanical changes so often amenable to manipulation.

These pathological changes should be invariably borne in mind in history taking, in general and local examination, as also in investigation of the patient.

They are discussed in detail in Chapter 8, particularly under general and specific contraindications to vertebral manipulation. It is stressed that meticulous adherence to the principles of manipulation is what makes it so very safe a clinical procedure.

The conditions of particular interest and importance for the clinician are rheumatoid arthritis, the seronegative arthritides, Scheuermann's disease, polymyalgia rheumatica, benign and malignant neoplasms, and non-reversible nerve damage.

Generally speaking, vertebral manipulation is most likely to prove helpful in the absence of demonstrable pathological changes, though often in spite of them – provided there is no contraindication.

8
Why and why not – indications and contraindications

This chapter is taken very largely from *Musculoskeletal Medicine, the Spine*[10].

Indication for manipulation

The prime indication for manipulation is the discovery of a painful segmental disorder (PSD). This is identified by taking an adequate history and by local examination of the back, as described in Chapter 11 (in addition to orthopaedic or neurological examination).

Skin pinching – anterior and posterior – alerts the examiner to the possibility of a PSD.

Localized areas of increased muscle tone suggest guarding of subjacent structures – which may be malfunctioning.

The sagittal pressure test seeks confirmation of malfunction by inducing passive sagittal movement of mobile segments, relative to their immediate neighbours. It suggests the level of malfunction but crudely.

The spinous process lateral pressure test is somewhat similar to the sagittal test but seeks to provoke passive rotation of mobile segments. Thus, it complements the sagittal test but particularly stresses tissues which restrict rotation, thus giving confirmation of the previous test and sometimes adding an indication of which side is affected.

Trigger points (together with tender points) discovered on palpation, are manifestations of referred tenderness: they suggest malfunction in the likely region of their origin. This may be distant from their site of perception.

Posterior joint tenderness, commonly accompanied by guarding, suggests the site of origin of a PSD. It does not commonly provide a diagnosis but it indicates the site to which ANY local therapy should be directed.

Contraindications to manipulation

These are divided into three groups: general clinical, specific clinical and technical.

The general clinical contraindications are as follows:

1. Recent bony fracture, which is elicited from the history.

2. Neoplasm, which is discovered from the history or orthodox examination, with or without investigations, and is most commonly secondary and derived from primary lesions of the breast, lung, kidney, prostate or thyroid.

3. Inflammatory diseases, such as Scheuermann's disease, ankylosing spondylitis or polymyalgia rheumatica.

4. Vascular conditions.

5. Osteoporosis (but remember that the gentleness of the appropriate techniques modifies the importance of this item). There can be no place in orthodox medicine for vigorous vertebral manipulation, whether performed under general anaesthesia or not.

The specific clinical contraindications, again several, are as follows:

1. Rheumatoid arthritis of the neck, because of the vulnerability of the dens and the transverse ligaments, resulting in risk of injury to the spinal cord.

2. Vertebral artery insufficiency, because of the possibility of occlusion of the blood supply to the circle of Willis by kinking the vertebral arteries. The diagnosis of insufficiency must be made on the history of drop attacks or postural vertigo, as testing for patency/occlusion has been shown to be a possible cause of disaster[34].

3. Grisel's syndrome, in which a child with a sore throat may develop a weakness of the transverse or alar ligaments, which may persist for several weeks after the infection has abated, is a contraindication for the same reason as rheumatoid arthritis of the neck.

4. Cervical, thoracic or lumbar myelopathy, as revealed by orthodox clinical history and examination; in particular, sphincter problems and saddle anaesthesia.

The over-riding contraindication to manipulation (and the one which throws serious doubt on the safety of manipulation under general anaesthesia) is when setting up the patient for manipulation causes appreciable pain.

There are NO technical contraindications to manipulation of the spine. The decision is simply to manipulate, or not to manipulate!

Dangers

There are approximately 3000–4000 manipulators in the UK alone. Even at as few as 6 per day each, this means 5 500 000 vertebral manipulations per annum!

The number of disasters reported since 1945 remains IN SINGLE FIGURES, which gives an incidence of reported disasters of 1:600 000. In spite of the views offered by a minority of the profession[8]:

MANIPULATION IS CLEARLY A *VERY* SAFE PROCEDURE!

9
What do you see? – Common presentations

The variety of presentation of musculoskeletal problems is derived largely from the twin phenomena of referred pain and referred tenderness.

Pain referred from the cervical spine

Pain may be referred rostrally, to the head, sometimes mimicking migraine or other head pain, but also to the face, mimicking ENT, dental or ophthalmological problems. (Remember Maigne's eyebrow test[10,47].)

Pain may be referred caudally, more often in the posterior distribution of the nerve, most often to the suprascapular and interscapular regions. Alternatively, it may be referred to the upper limb, including the shoulder, elbow, wrist and hand[10,36,47]. Apparent tennis elbow, golfer's elbow and carpal tunnel syndrome may prove to have a vertebral origin, solely or in combination with local causes.

It may be referred caudally and anteriorly, mimicking coronary ischaemia[48].

Whatever its segmental distribution, it may be diffuse, unilateral or bilateral, and it may be associated with numbness (both ulnar and radial) and also with reduced brachial reflexes, spastic gait and even reduced leg reflexes[36].

Failure to seek local physical signs in the neck may result in inappropriate treatment of brachial or thoracic pain.

Pain referred from the thoracic spine

This is particularly common, arising around T4 and presenting as anterior chest pain – 20% in Fossgreen's series[48] – approximately the same incidence as negative ECGs in the routine investigation of possible coronary ischaemic pain.

There is surgical evidence that abdominal pain may be of thoracic vertebral origin, most commonly between T6 and T12[49]. There is similar evidence derived from injection techniques[50].

Buttock, inguinal, scrotal, crural and sciatic referral may give rise to similar diagnostic difficulties.

Maigne's work provides evidence of a possible anatomical explanation of such apparent referral, in that he has shown that the T12–L2 posterior rami extend to the buttock, crossing the iliac crest, and they may suffer entrapment on emergence through the lumbar fascia[45]. This may be relieved by manipulation or by injection but it may require surgical relief. It has been estimated that up to 60% of buttock

26

pain is due to the latter cause. It is worth while remembering this when considering pain in the region of the sacroiliac joints.

Pain referred from the lumbar source

True sciatica is unlikely to be missed, but buttock, inguinal, scrotal and crural pain may arise in the lumbar spine as well as in the lower thoracic spine. Sciatica does NOT necessarily indicate a disc protrusion, whatever the putative level.

Pain of visceral origin

Confusion may arise from the fact that pain of cardiac, pulmonary, diaphragmatic, abdominal or pelvic origin may present in precisely the same sites as does referred pain of vertebral origin.

Pain of rheumatological origin

Ankylosing spondylitis, the seronegative arthropathies, polymyalgia rheumatica and painful osteoporosis may, of course, further confuse the scene.

Conclusion

Another difficulty in differentiation between these possible causes of pain lies in the likelihood of coexistence of two or more causes, coupled with the possibility of summation of symptoms.

The vital lesson to be learned is that almost ANY pain MAY have a vertebral origin, in toto or in part, and that this means two things:

1. All clinicians should be aware of this fact.

2. Local examination of the spine is a necessary part of clinical assessment of almost ALL painful complaints. For this reason, *it now demands to be incorporated as a part of the undergraduate syllabus – on wholly orthodox grounds, rather than as a result of any unorthodox claims*.

As might be expected, there was unanimous agreement in the workshop on this point, although considerable discussion took place before this was reached.

10
How do you assess cases? – Case analysis

The term case analysis is used, rather than diagnosis, because of the unpredictability of the twin phenomena of referred pain and referred tenderness, and because nociceptor systems are present in many sites, and therefore, 'in the great majority of cases we do not know the tissue or tissues from which back pain is originating, or the cause of that pain'. This last statement may upset some, and it demands consideration from the points of view of both history and examination. This chapter is taken very largely from *Musculoskeletal Medicine, the Spine*[10].

As far as history is concerned:

1. The phenomenon of referred pain means that the site of perception of pain is not necessarily of diagnostic significance and indeed is frequently misleading.

2. The 'hornet's nest' of physiological activity to be found at all levels of the neuraxis, periphery, dorsal horn, EMAS and cerebral cortex, means that symptoms are inevitably subject to modification on this count alone.

As far as examination is concerned:

1. The phenomenon of referred tenderness mirrors that of referred pain.

2. The 'hornet's nest' referred to above is as applicable to physical signs as it is to symptoms. Physical signs may vary from time to time in response to numerous uncontrollable factors.

On scientific grounds, *physiological parameters cannot therefore be legitimately used in case analysis as a means of measurement of pain.*

However, the physiological phenomena that may or may not accompany pain can, with certain limitations, be used in case analysis without causing orthodox offence.

In this system of case analysis, primacy is allocated to behavioural indices because these are objective and thus can be agreed by all clinicians, whatever their discipline, and because they can be measured to a known degree of accuracy. This greatly simplifies the complex question of patient assessment and avoids the difficulties inherent in subject report. Patients always edit their histories, always in accordance with their understanding of their problem, often in response to what they assume the doctor will expect and occasionally for perceived personal advantage. A selection of these criteria is used, in the knowledge that no single response channel can ever be an adequate method of evaluation, but that, in aggregate, they afford the clinician a practical basis for case analysis and subsequent decisions regarding management.

History

Reference to the case analysis record sheet will show that routine administrative data need no description. They are followed by a list of contraindications to manipulation which has a dual purpose: first, as a checklist for the busy clinician, second as a defence against possible complaint or litigation. The history record is divided into three parts: patient report (deliberately curtailed), activities of daily living (offering a broad choice of indices) and pain behaviour. Three columns provide for entries on three dates, entered in the uppermost boxes.

Patient report

The site and radiation of pain are entered (in left or right boxes) labelled by the segmental reference and whether in the anterior or posterior radiation (e.g. C4A or C5P).

The reported intensity of pain is recorded as mild, moderate or severe, entered by +, + + or + + +. Its duration is entered in shorthand (e.g. 1/7, 3/52, 5/12, etc.).

Factors causing pain to worsen or improve are entered in words.

Pins and needles and numbness must be sought. They are not always volunteered by the patient. In particular, the patient must be asked about saddle anaesthesia and disturbances of micturition (raising the question of sacral root compression). This is entered by the same coding as is used for the site and radiation of pain. Also, he must be asked whether he has had symptoms suggesting basilar artery insufficiency (giddiness etc. on looking up), and a history of disturbance of gait raises the possibility of myelopathy; no special place is provided for these to be entered but their importance is such as to warrant a large entry demanding attention!

Activities of daily living

A selection of these is included, as they offer a guide to the disability suffered without recourse to emotive symptoms. Here, in each case, disability is entered as being mild, moderate or severe, using +, + + or + + +.

Pain behaviour

Pill taking is entered in words (e.g. codeine × 2 qds). Other treatments are entered in words. The space provided may not be sufficient, in which case overflow will occur!

Hours in bed in the 24 may be significant, entered by a simple figure.

The duration of forced absenteeism from work may be pertinent, and this is entered in figures (e.g. 5/7, 2/52, 3/12).

Pending or current litigation again may be of significance, and a positive reply is readily entered by a tick.

Previous episodes

In the case of recurrences, the last two episodes are entered as indicated.

Relevant medical history

Provision is made on the form for this, and details of what factors are important are discussed under indications and contraindications (Chapter 8). Entry is made in words or private shorthand.

The final entry, under 'affect', allows discreet comment to be made on the suitability of the patient for various therapies.

Conclusion

The practical features of this system of case analysis are:

1. It is based on the relevant anatomical, physiological, psychological and pathological facts, as they are currently understood.

2. It thereby avoids dogma, as baneful an influence in musculoskeletal medicine as in other fields.

3. Whatever its acknowledged shortcomings, it provides a *rational* basis for clinical assessment and management, sufficient in most cases to permit a therapeutic decision to be made, without recourse to unorthodox or frankly invalid hypotheses.

4. It is brief enough to be of use to every clinician, particularly the general practitioner. General practice is, of course, where the great majority of these cases is best treated, from start to finish.

5. Because it is founded on currently valid scientific considerations, it will inevitably be subject to modification in the light of further knowledge and understanding. For the same reason, it will remain wholly acceptable to the orthodox in its modified form. As such, it may be seen as a suitable base for an introductory course in musculoskeletal medicine.

6. The case analysis sheet provides a checklist for the clinician which aims at:

   (a) Being sufficiently comprehensive for its purpose.

   (b) Affording comparability of data from different observers, thus allowing collective research.

7. While a sheet of this size and complexity looks rather daunting, this is, in practice, somewhat misleading, as, with a very little experience in its use, it is quicker to enter the data than writing it out in longhand. It is also quicker to extract data for follow-up or research purposes. It is also well suited to computer adaptation.

   Local examination is dealt with in the following chapter.

MUSCULOSKELETAL CASE ANALYSIS SHEET

Patient's name...Serial No:.......................

Address ....

....Phone ....

Date of birth   /   /   Male:.............Female.........Insurance.......................

Contraindications: Fractures....... Neoplasm........ Scheuermann........ A/spondylitis......
Polymyalgia........ Osteoporosis........ Rh.A. of neck........ Basilar insuff........ Grisel......
Myelopathy........ Sphincter problems........ Saddle anaesthesia........

HISTORY – Present episode

Subject report	/ /		/ /		/ /	
	L	R	L	R	L	R
Pain – Site						
Radiation						
Intensity						
Duration						
Worsened by						
Improved by						

Altered sensation

	L	R	L	R	L	R
P & N						
Numbness						

Activities of daily living

	L	R	L	R	L	R
Hoovering						
Bedmaking						
Ablutions						
Cooking						
Ironing						
Putting on socks						
Shopping						
Gardening						
Sports						
Sitting at desk						
Other work						
Road/rail travel						
Air travel						

Pain behaviour

	L	R	L	R	L	R
Pill taking habit						
Other treatments						
Hours in bed per 24						
Forced absenteeism						
Litigation pending						

Previous episodes

Year ....Site ....Duration in days.............weeks ....months ....
Therapy ....Outcome ....
Year ....Site ....Duration in days.............weeks ....months ....
Therapy ....Outcome ....
Relevant medical history ....
....
Affect ....

Examined
Stance (posture)

	/ /	/ /	/ /

Global movements

	Initial	Follow-up 1	Follow-up 2

Cervical

SB — FI — SB   Rot — Rot   EX (Initial)

SB — FI — SB   Rot — Rot   EX (Follow-up 1)

SB — FI — SB   Rot — Rot   EX (Follow-up 2)

Lumbar

SB — FI — SB   Rot — Rot   EX (Initial)

SB — FI — SB   Rot — Rot   EX (Follow-up 1)

SB — FI — SB   Rot — Rot   EX (Follow-up 2)

Traditional signs

	/ /		/ /		/ /	
	L	R	L	R	L	R
Biceps reflex						
Supinator reflex						
Triceps reflex						
Knee reflex						
Ankle reflex						
Plantar reflex						
Straight leg raising						
Altered sensation						
Additional signs						

Local signs

Skin tenderness						
Trigger points						
Local guarding						
Sagittal SPP						
Lateral SPP						
Tender Z-A joints						
Iliac separation						
Iliac compression						
Sacral pressure						

Invesigations ....

THERAPY

11
What are you looking for?

It is important to remember that the local examination presented here is an *addition* to the clinical examination taught in medical school: an addition which, in conjunction with an adequate history, enables the clinician to make rational management decisions in the very common absence of a valid diagnosis. Its basis is wholly acceptable to the orthodox. This chapter is taken very largely from *Musculoskeletal Medicine, the Spine*[10].

The structured data recording, which is an integral part of it, is important for two reasons: first, because it permits rapid and detailed recall of information at some future date, second because it enables the research-minded to make valid comparisons between different observers. Further, it offers a bonus in that it also affords the busy clinician another useful checklist!

Traditional examination

As in the case of recording the history, the data sheet shown on the preceding pages provides three columns for the recording of dates of attendance, relating to posture and movement, again entered for the remainder of the examination record.

Posture

This is included (whether it has great significance or not) recorded in writing and symbols, as shown. As this is so widely variable in the absence of symptoms, only relatively gross deviations are recorded. Its aetiological relationship to pain remains unclear. Its chief value lies in monitoring progress, rather than in a move towards diagnosis. The serial changes in posture which constitute gait are excluded from this basic syllabus, as being clinically irrelevant and confusing to the novice; also as being anathema to the serious doctor. (See Chapter 19.)

Global movements

These also are included largely for their value in monitoring response to therapy. They have little proven relevance to diagnosis. Assessment is deliberately crude because it is not possible to identify the normal range of movement clinically (see

Chapter 13), thereby rendering it impossible to identify the abnormal. For this reason, a reduction in what seems likely to be normal is recorded somewhat crudely as slight, moderate or severe, using the opposite movement as a rough guide; and this is entered on the data sheet by one, two or three short lines across any of the six lines of the diagram. This simple method of recording saves a great deal of time; it is borrowed from Maigne[47].

As an extra use of this diagram, in the case of any movement being restricted by pain, the degree of pain caused by that movement is recorded (again crudely) as being mild, moderate or severe, marking these by one, two or three crosses on the appropriate line.

In the interests of simplicity, diagrams are available for the cervical and lumbar regions only, one for each of the dates entered above them, as it is by no means certain that it would be useful to provide also for the thoracic region.

Tendon reflexes

These are an intrinsic part of traditional examination, and they are recorded only when clearly increased, decreased or absent. These are entered by use of +, − or 0 in the appropriate box. Normal findings are not entered, as this is wasteful of time.

Straight leg raising

On the other hand, in this case, the approximate angle (degrees) raised from the horizontal on either side is entered. Once again, contrary to some teaching, this is likely to be of value in monitoring therapeutic progress, rather than as a diagnostic sign. The identification of normal range is extremely difficult, wide variations being common.

Altered sensation

In the case of altered sensation, use is made of segmental labelling, in the knowledge that it bears little diagnostic significance; *it is no more than a topographical indicator*. This is entered in either the left or the right box, using the segmental reference, and adding A or P to indicate whether an alteration was found anteriorly or posteriorly.

Additional signs

This space is left for use where a further sign is thought to be of value by the individual clinician.

Local clinical tests

These are all unoriginal and are presented in terms as explicit and orthodox as possible, avoiding the jargon that has so often clouded them in the past. They are very largely adapted from Maigne[47]. They must be sought anteriorly as well as posteriorly. (It is important to remind students that pain and tenderness of spinal origin can be referred to the anterior chest and abdominal wall, a fact potentially confusing.)

Further, in view of the difficulties emphasized already, local examination *must* be comprehensive. The whole spine should always be examined.

Although only four tests are used in the neck (for reasons which will become apparent), two further tests are added for most of the spine, and there are three more applicable to the pelvis.

Skin pinching

This is a test for tenderness of the skin and subcutaneous tissues. The examiner raises a fold of skin at paired sites either side of the midline and pinches as nearly symmetrically as he can, asking the patient to report any differences in sensation between left and right. In practice, for most of the spine, he rolls the skinfold caudally, thus ensuring that he does not miss a potentially tender area. Because of the phenomenon of referred tenderness, this must be done widely, both posteriorly and anteriorly. Regarding the cervical spine, the face and anterior neck must be remembered, and the eyebrow test of Maigne[47].

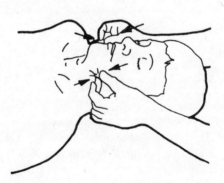

Anterior skin pinching – facial

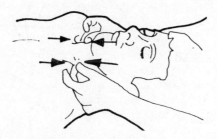

Anterior skin pinching – cervical

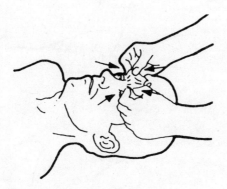

Anterior skin pinching – eyebrow (Maigne)

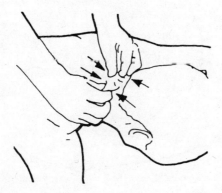

Posterior skin pinching – cervical

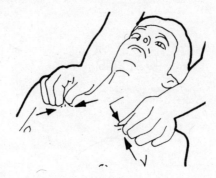

Anterior skin pinching – thoracic

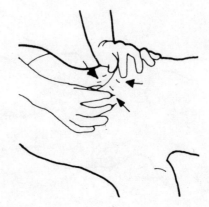

Posterior skin pinching – thoracic

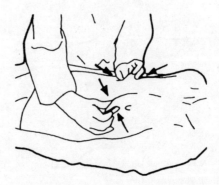

Anterior skin pinching – thoracic

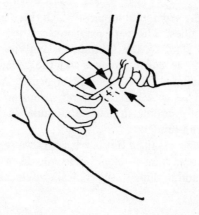

Posterior skin pinching – lumbar

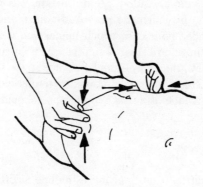

Anterior skin pinching – lumbar

Frequently, the examiner will observe a difference in thickness of the skinfold between the two sides at the level the patient reports tenderness. This difference may be eliminated on resolution of the tenderness. There is currently no valid explanation for this phenomenon. A positive finding does *not* indicate the segmental level of dysfunction.

Recording of a positive result of this test is made as shown (e.g. in the right box, C3A indicates a positive test on the right at the third cervical level, in the anterior distribution). It must be remembered that the segmental label is nothing more than a topographical indicator.

Muscle guarding

This test seeks to identify segmental levels at which there is a difference in muscle tone between the two sides. The paraspinal musculature is palpated bilaterally, from the base of the skull to the sacrum, asking the patient to report any tenderness. It is easier to do this in the neck with the patient supine, while the rest of the spine may be palpated either standing or prone. A positive finding, while clearly primarily subjective, is well known to physicians and generally accepted by them, as in the case of guarding in acute abdominal pathology. This finding is commonly associated with tenderness.

Recording of a positive result of this test is as shown (e.g. C5P in the left box). There is no virtue in attempting to identify the muscle or measure the degree of increased tone – these add nothing to the clinical usefulness of the test.

Trigger points

Palpation also elicits tenderness in trigger points. Since these may be found widely, they must be sought equally widely. A distinction was made in the workshop between trigger points, in which the provoked pain is radiated distant from the trigger point, and tender points, in which tenderness is elicited at the point of pressure. Clearly, these are two different phenomena, although, from a therapeutic point of view, they may often be treated in the same way.

Recording the presence of trigger points or tender points employs the same principle; the segmental label is a rough topographical guide only.

Segmental sagittal pressure

This test seeks to elicit pain on applying a midline sagittal force to the spinous processes at successive segmental levels. It serves to implicate either the vertebra to which it is applied, or the various joints above and below. Since the spinous processes in the cervical spine (except for that of C7) are so deep and small as to be in practice difficult to identify with any accuracy, this test is inapplicable to the cervical region. Of course, many more joints are moved by this test than those immediately adjacent to the vertebra pressed upon but the force and resultant movement are concentrated to a considerable extent in sequence at each segmental level examined.

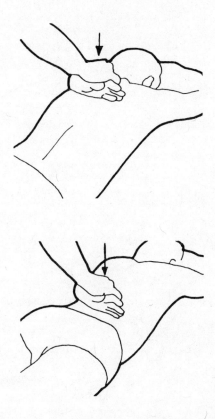

Pain produced by this test is entered across the L/R dividing line, using the crude segmental level, or on either side in the case of the pain being provoked unilaterally.

Lateral spinous process pressure

This test produces a forced rotation of successive vertebrae, performed by pressing with the thumbs on the lateral aspect of each spinous process, alternately to the left and the right. Once more, it involves a *minimum* of *all* the joints between the vertebra pressed upon and its two neighbours, but many more joints must be affected, so rendering it wholly non-specific. Again, this test is inapplicable in the cervical spine, owing to the small size and deep situation of the spinous processes.

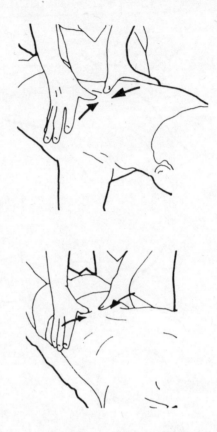

Pain produced by this test is entered in the left or right box according to the direction of pressure, rather than the site of pain. Remember that pressing the spinous process to the patient's left produces a clockwise rotation of that vertebra between its neighbours, and vice versa.

Zygoapophyseal joint tenderness

This test seeks to reveal any tenderness there may be of the posterior vertebral joint capsules and adjacent structures, in an attempt to locate more accurately the site of origin of the pain. The examiner presses firmly over the joints at each segmental level in turn and asks the patient to report tenderness at any site. The joints lie at each segmental level, approximately one (patient's) finger's breadth to either side of the midline. Apart from its use in determining a possible site of dysfunction, this test is of value in that it may reveal the potentially most suitable site for any local treatment (e.g. injection). It is more specific than the previous two tests, in that it gives a clearer indication of the side as well as the segmental

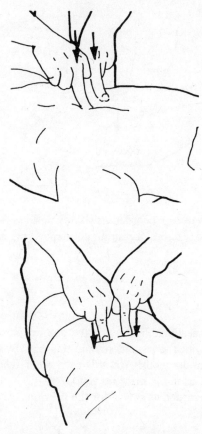

level. In the neck, it is well to perform this test with the patient supine, as the muscles are thereby more relaxed and the articular pillars more readily palpated.

Recording is as shown: mild, moderate or severe pain being recorded as +, + + or + + + in the appropriate box.

Iliac separation

This test is of relatively infrequent value in drawing attention to a possible strain of the anterior sacroiliac ligaments. With the patient supine, press sharply and simultaneously with the heel of each hand on the anterior superior iliac spines, the direction of thrust being down and laterally. In view of the comments on pelvic anatomy in Chapter 18, the temptation to interpret the result of this test too literally should be resisted.

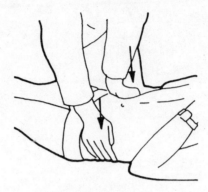

Pain provoked by this test is recorded as shown, with +, + + or + + + either in one box or the other, or across the midline, depending upon the site of pain provoked.

Iliac compression

To stress the posterior sacroiliac ligaments, the anterior superior iliac spines are used again; once more with the patient supine, this time by pressing sharply with the heels of the hands simultaneously towards each other. The same limitations on interpretation apply here as in the previous test.

A positive result is recorded as shown for the previous two tests.

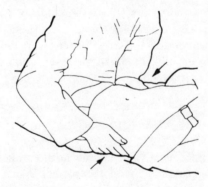

Sacral sagittal pressure test

This test may be used to confirm an impression derived from either of the last two tests; it involves a rapid short-amplitude vertical thrust with the heel of the hand on the sacrum, with the patient prone.

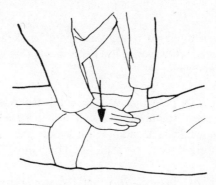

It is easiest to apply this thrust reinforced by the other hand. A similar test, 'springing' the symphysis pubis, adds little to clinical assessment.

Recording is as shown for the previous three tests.

It will be noted that no attempt is made to identify any specific position or movement of the pelvic components, as this is not necessary for the identification of the site to which local therapy is to be directed, and it reopens discussion regarding questions which remain hypothetical and currently inappropriate to *basic* musculoskeletal medicine. (See Chapter 18.)

Investigations

According to Haslock, special investigations are surprisingly seldom required in musculoskeletal practice. Such investigations as are from time to time regarded as necessary by the clinician include the following:

Conventional radiology	Thermography
Myelography	Electromyography
Radiculography	Discography
Electronystagmography/cupulography	Scintigraphy
Epidurography	Radioactive isotope studies
Ultrasonography	Magnetic resonance imaging
Transverse axial tomography	Erythrocyte sedimentation rate
Serum urea estimation	Tomography
Interosseous spinal venography	Serum uric acid estimation
Vertebral artery angiography	Rose Waaler test
Intervertebral disc manometry	Latex test

This list is not intended to be comprehensive, rather it is offered to stress the very considerable number of tests which may be relevant in individual cases. A few demand comment.

Conventional radiology

1. Attempts have been made to relate back pain to skeletal defects, be they congenital or acquired. However, it has been shown that many different defects exist without causing pain[51].

2. Just as the detection by palpation of segmental hyper- and hypomobility has been used to diagnose spinal lesions and monitor their treatment, so has conventional radiology. In fact, radiological hyper- and hypomobility and their responses to manipulative treatment have never been conclusively demonstrated.

    The fact that it has been shown that the over-riding of zygoapophyseal joints of 3 mm in the middle of the cervical spine and 3.5 mm at the level of L5 and S1 was not detectable on routine X-rays indicates the difficulty of such endeavours[52]. This over-riding also affords the clinician an important safety factor, which will be discussed under posterior joint injections. (See Appendix 6.)

3. There is no positive correlation between degenerative changes shown by conventional radiology and pain. Yet all doctors will know of the patient who has been told by another clinician that, because of degenerative changes in his spine, shown radiologically, his back pain is fixed and there is little or nothing anyone can do for him. In view of what has just been said, this is simply not so.

Radiology and a number of other scanning techniques are dealt with rather more fully in Chapter 12.

Conclusions

Together, and as an addition to orthodox examination, search for the local physical signs described permits the clinician to make a rational decision as to management, in the absence of a formal diagnosis.

While it may at first sight appear complicated, this method of data recording is in practice very simple. As already stated, it acts as a checklist and lends itself to collective research. More important, however, with the minimum of experience, it is in fact quicker to enter than are equivalent longhand notes, and it is also quicker and easier to read.

Finally, there is nothing used in this method which is not immediately acceptable to the orthodox medical profession. In my view, there is no logical hindrance to local examination becoming an integral part of orthodox clinical practice.

12
The place of radiology, CAT scans, ultrasound and magnetic resonance imaging

When are radiology, etc. indicated? When relevant and necessary evidence is not otherwise available. How do they help? By any of the following means:

1. Exclusion of pathology.
2. Confirmation of clinical findings.
3. For legal and insurance considerations.

Indications

1. When there is no real clue available from the history.
2. When no confirmation is forthcoming from orthodox or local examination.
3. On unexpected failure therapeutically.
4. At the patient's request – for reassurance of the patient.
5. For legal and insurance purposes – for the protection of the doctor as much as for the benefit of the patient.

Value to the clinician

1. They may help in the decision whether or not to manipulate. But it must be remembered that gross changes are easy to identify whereas minor changes are often more important.

2. Specialist advice may be very helpful, but one must always learn the specialist's language! The radiologist may use his own special jargon, not always immediately familiar! Commonly, radiologists appear to disagree simply because they are using different forms of jargon.

3. It is worth preserving a certain humility in observing X-rays etc. when one is fortunate enough to see them for oneself.

Limitations

1. From a technical point of view, remember that normal pictures do NOT necessarily mean normal state or normal function.

2. From a professional point of view, remember also that abnormal pictures do NOT always mean abnormal state or abnormal function.

3. Remember the inevitable time-lag in the appearance of radiologically abnormal signs, and also that even very accurate measurement of observed factors may be irrelevant or misleading if these have been shown to vary widely and randomly in the asymptomatic subject.

Routine

1. Identification of the patient. It is important to ensure that the picture is of the particular patient, and that it is the most up-to-date available! This may seem elementary, but mistakes are made, and these can have far-reaching results: in choice of therapy, in results and in litigation.

2. Posture – AP – observe rotation, side-bending or scoliosis.
   Lateral – is the spine 'straight', extended, flexed or showing spondylolisthesis?
   Oblique views – if indicated.

3. Congential – look for cervical ribs, pars defects or spina bifida.

4. Intervertebral spaces – observe reduction of spaces in degenerative disc disease.

5. Sclerosis – in degenerative disease, rheumatoid and TB.

6. Osteophytosis – in degenerative disease – intervertebral/apophyseal/ foraminal.

7. Porosis, which may be – generalized, senile or hormonal.
   localized – Ca, TB, rheumatoid,
   Scheuermann's disease.

8. Cortical breaches – as may arise in the following: Ca, sarcoma, rheumatoid and odd arthritides.

9. Interpedicular expansion – may indicate intramedullary tumours.

10. Ankylosing spondylitis. Again, physical signs are likely to precede radiological signs.

CAT scans

1. These are more accurate than X-ray, plain or myelogram or radiculogram.
2. They are earlier in picking up localized porosis, etc.
3. They give useful pictures of soft tissues.
4. They involve greater irradiation to the patient.
5. They are of far greater cost.

Ultrasound scans

1. These give variable results – excellent if well performed.
2. They are not so widely available.
3. They are 'user-friendly' in that they have no noxious effects.

Magnetic resonance imaging

1. This produces magnificent imaging.
2. It also involves enormous cost.
3. It is extremely unpleasant for the patient – very claustrophobic and quite deafening.

Final thoughts

1. Whenever possible, it is best to try to make your own decisions regarding the significance of your findings – then refer to the report or ask for help from your radiologist!

2. In view of the prevalence of referral of pain and tenderness and the common incidence of asymptomatic disc bulges, a better view of a bulge is not of consistent benefit to the patient!

3. Most patients with pain of vertebral origin are seen early.

Twelve pertinent facts currently valid

1. Every serious hypothesis DEMANDS adequate testing.

2. Valid testing reveals an hypothesis to be TRUE or FALSE.

3. Valid new evidence DEMANDS reassessment of an hypothesis.

4. Data MUST be drawn from an adequate sample of a defined population.

5. Statistical analysis DEMANDS measurable indices.

6. Analysis MUST be statistically significant to warrant change of belief.

7. Any hypothesis shown to be false MUST be abandoned – publicly.

8. Subjective impressions are NOT measurable.

9. Therefore subjective impressions are NOT admissable, (see 5).

10. NO vertebra is perfectly bilaterally symmetrical.

11. NO TWO vertebrae are identical.

12. Range of vertebral movement in the asymptomatic subject varies WIDELY and RANDOMLY

    a) at serial segmental levels in the individual.
    b) at the same segmental levels between individuals.

Failure to adapt musculoskeletal teaching to these twelve FACTS GUARANTEES non-acceptance by the orthodox medical profession.

PART II

Part I of this small book presents a simple, scientifically acceptable basis upon which vertebral manipulation may be taught and practised in safety, with reasonable expectation of therapeutic success and without recourse to controversial hypothesis. Presented in this light, it is acceptable to the orthodox medical profession, and it must be stressed that (contrary to some beliefs) coupled with a quite short practical course, it is sufficient for the novice to make use of this potentially valuable therapeutic option. However, because of the widespread promotion of some of these controversial hypotheses, and because their adoption by a number of doctors has been in some measure responsible for vertebral manipulation being regarded as a part of 'fringe medicine', it is necessary now to consider the main ones with a view to eliminating them from basic teaching.

This is not to say that they should be summarily abandoned by their proponents; rather that they should be reserved for those who find them a help *after assimilation of the scientific basis*, and also for those who wish to pursue the possibility of establishing a scientifically acceptable basis for them. This seems a proper research goal, wholly compatible with orthodox thinking. However, as will be seen from Part II, as yet this has not been achieved.

13
Joint mobility

Before considering this subject in any detail, it has to be appreciated that (in the absence of breakage of bone) the smallest movable spinal unit is the mobile segment of Junghanns, and that, clinically, this is of theoretical interest only as numerous segments move at any one time, actively or passively (whether diagnostically or therapeutically), each of their constituent joints moving in a different manner and to a different degree.

This is a subject of interest to some doctors and many physiotherapists, while it is one of the cornerstones of osteopathic diagnosis. For the doctor seriously interested in musculoskeletal medicine, it has to be scrutinized with some care. Its exclusion from the basic musculoskeletal syllabus (see the Introduction and also Appendix 4) is deliberate, but this demands further explanation if a scientific approach is to be maintained.

Rather than approaching joint mobility directly, it is more realistic first to discuss joint blockage and joint stiffness. Many osteopaths, chiropractors and some doctors believe in reduced mobility being the core of articular dysfunction (and sometimes many other problems)[53,54]. This argument is seen to be scientifically fallible, as the identification of normal spinal joint mobility in a clinical setting is seldom possible; in which case it must be *impossible to identify the abnormal* with any certainty[10,36]. The truth is that the range of movement of the spinal joints varies widely and without proven correlation with other factors.

For many years the analogy of the jammed drawer has been used to illustrate the concept of the blocked joint. It may be found profitable to examine this analogy in some detail. A drawer is, in plan, a rigid, usually oblong object, designed to slide between the parallel sides of the space in the rigid chest made to accept it. The outside transverse measurements of the drawer (a) must be less than the inside transverse measurement of its 'slot' in the carcass of the chest (b). The deliberate difference between these two measurements is the play allowed (c) to enable the drawer to slide in and out (Figure 1).

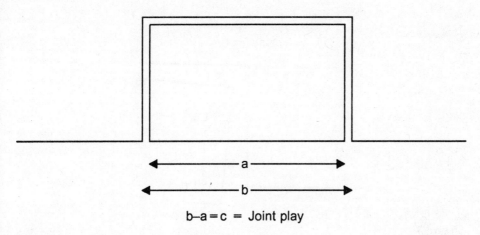

$$b-a = c = \text{Joint play}$$

Figure 1

The drawer may be jammed (in its horizontal plane) in one way only: when it is rotated about an axis perpendicular to that plane so that its oblique measurement (d) approximates to the transverse measurement of the 'slot' (b) when the slack has been taken up. The resultant jamming is between some point on one side of the carcass in contact with the posterior corner of the drawer on that side, and the opposite anterior corner of the carcass in contact with some point on the opposite side of the drawer. Clearly a sharp small-amplitude tap, as indicated by the arrow in Figure 2, is likely to free the drawer.

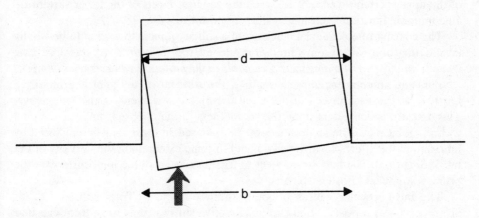

Figure 2

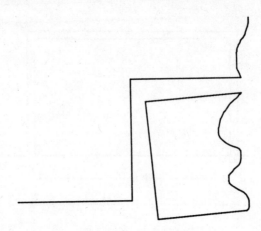

Figure 3

Of course, the analogy breaks down because the drawer is contained between the two rigid 'jaws' of the chest with which it articulates both on the left and on the right. Thus it represents two paired joints, not one.

Take either of them in isolation and it is immediately clear that *no mechanical jamming or blockage can possibly take place* (Figure 3). Theoretically, such jamming might take place between a pair of joints, provided that their facets were, all four of them, parallel. But is this to be found in man's back? Happily for man, though sadly for the analogy, no! The nearest approach to this state is in the pairs of posterior vertebral joints of the lumbar spine, but, even here, the appreciable obliquity of their facets means that rotational mechanical jamming is impossible, the only mechanical block possible being found on forcing both the inferior facets of the upper vertebra ventrally between the superior facets of the lower vertebra – an admirable function, guarding against spondylolisthesis!

The concept of mechanical blockage of a solitary joint is thus seen to be wholly invalid, that of a pair of joints pretty far fetched. *It is difficult to see, therefore, how it can form any part of a diagnosis acceptable to the orthodox, whoever champions it.*

Pursuing another engineering analogy, the stiffness of any joint is primarily a function of the friction caused in it on attempted movement, active or passive. This, in turn, is dependent upon the smoothness of the opposed surfaces, coupled with the joint play. The smoothness of the opposed surfaces may be enhanced by lubrication, the effect of which will depend to some extent upon the viscosity of the lubricating fluid. The long-term effect of friction is wear of the joint surfaces – the prime component of osteoarthrosis.

The intra-articular causes of joint stiffness are few. Total stiffness means arthrodesis or ankylosis – bony union. Relative stiffness may arise from capsular fibrosis secondary to arthritic changes (possibly accentuated by ligamentous overgrowth) or haemarthrosis. Roughened articular cartilage may cause stiffness only in the absence of synovial effusion, as the effusion counteracts this effect by increasing joint play and separating the roughened surfaces (though at the same time causing stiffness by putting the capsule under strain). There is no other intra-articular structure which can cause stiffness of a joint, other than by increase in viscosity of the synovial fluid. It is extremely doubtful whether a loose body in a joint mechanically blocks its movement – it may give rise to pain (provoking neuromuscular changes outside the joint) but there is no evidence of which I am aware which shows that the mechanism of any restriction appearing to result from an intra-articular loose body does indeed lie inside the joint.

The extra-articular causes of stiffness of a joint are again few. Bony abnormality may restrict the range of joint movement by its physical obstruction to approximation of the two relevant bony shafts. The development of osteophytes may similarly restrict the range of movement of a joint, from which it may be deduced that 'normal' joint range is something likely to lessen with the process of ageing; there can be no such thing as identifiable, absolute normality of range.

Oedema of the joint capsule, or other changes in fluid content, will render it less pliable and thereby stiffen a joint. Shortening of the fibres of the capsule, for example in post-traumatic fibrosis, will restrict the possible range of movement, although perhaps without rendering it stiff within its new limits. Similarly, fibrosis in the supporting ligaments will restrict range of movement, while conversely excessive laxity will permit a range of movement greater than may be natural, thus allowing the capsule to be overstretched. None of these possibilities is rapidly reversible, so that none may explain the often immediate restoration of pain-free movement range common subsequent to manipulation.

Review of the neuromuscular literature reveals that, complex though the nervous control systems may be, it is the changing balance of tension or tone in a number of muscles (agonists, antagonists and synergists) which determines either the movement of a joint or its non-movement[55]. Again, there is no valid evidence of which I am aware in support of the suggestion that apparent articular stiffness commonly arises within a joint; it appears, in the great majority of cases, to be an extra-articular neuromuscular phenomenon. Terms like 'easy normal' range of joint movement and shifting 'movement barriers' can therefore do little but confuse the serious student of musculoskeletal medicine, at the same time antagonizing the sceptical. This concept has little to do with the joint.

It follows that anything that interferes with the neuromuscular control systems, including pain and numerous emotional factors, must contribute to both joint movement range and its lack, and to apparent joint stiffness.

Similarly, it is hard to imagine how a joint may be legitimately regarded as either blocked or intrinsically stiff. We are once again in the realm of fantasy. In view of the above facts, it is clear that to use vertebral joint mobility as a basis for specific diagnosis is scientifically unsound, and, indeed, there are three further reservations regarding the use of mobility tests in local examination:

1. They are almost entirely subjective, so that the sceptical will remain for ever fully entitled to their scepticism. They are not clinically measurable. This difficulty is in no way lessened by the employment of such hypothetical concepts as the 'movement' barrier: unproven and again solely reliant upon subjective impressions.

2. The 'normal' range of vertebral movement varies enormously, making its positive identification very difficult[56,57].

3. Despite a great deal of work world-wide, 'vertebral mobility is not fully understood'[55].

The chance of acceptance by the orthodox must recede with every resort to such hypothetical considerations. And, as has been seen in Chapters 10 and 11, there is no clinical necessity for this approach. Nonetheless, participants in the workshop remained divided on this question.

14
Bony position

The statement that a bone is out of place is commonly made. Indeed, this concept is fundamental for numerous practitioners. It is widely accepted by patients and also by some doctors, the therapeutic repositioning of bones being similarly widely accepted. On the other hand, it is also quite understandably the source of a considerable degree of dismissal by the orthodox medical profession. For this reason, this concept needs careful thought.

Before considering bony position at all, the serious doctor must remember three facts about the bones in question.

1. No vertebra is ever perfectly symmetrical[58].

2. Neither are any two vertebrae ever identical in form[58].

3. All vertebrae are subject to physiological structural changes with the passage of time; some, to a certain extent, predictable, some dependent upon nutritional or hormonal influences, with the addition of possible traumatic or pathological factors. After all, bone is a living structure.

Next it is necessary to consider the means available for clinical assessment of bony position, and their limitations.

1. Primarily this involves tactile sensation via the examiner's fingertips.

2. But the bony contours to be assessed lie deep to skin, subcutaneous tissues, fat, fascia and muscle, which must obscure their outline to a degree varying with the physical mass and current state of those tissues in each individual.

3. The greater the thickness of these soft tissues, the greater the pressure which needs to be exerted by the examining finger to reach an impression of bony contour.

4. The greater the degree of tension in the intervening muscles, the greater the pressure required to even find the bony prominences. And, of course, in the presence of pain or tenderness and resultant guarding, or of apprehension, that tension may be substantial.

57

5. Of far greater importance than the effort required, the greater the pressure exerted, the less delicate is the necessarily subjective sensory impression derived by the examiner from palpation. Useful mechanoceptive input from the examining finger is, after all, roughly inversely proportional to the pressure exerted on it.

Some may note that my reference to the asymmetry of vertebrae and their dissimilarity one from another is nearly fifty years old; it seems unlikely that human evolution will have altered man significantly in this short period! Neither has anybody shown this finding to be wrong. In view of the facts given above, it is clear that, as a result of the impossibility of clinically identifying normal position (and therefore also of abnormal position), the examiner's subjective impression of differences in 'knobbliness' between left and right can have little validity in proposing or supporting a positional diagnosis, even in the slender relaxed patient, while in the thick-set apprehensive patient with pain, such an impression has to be of *negligible* diagnostic significance. It is thus left to radiology or other scanning methods to make any sort of assessment of bony position, and there are grave doubts to be expressed as to the relevance of such observations. My comments on the bones themselves apply equally to any form of scanning. (See Chapter 12.)

Of course, vertebral malposition may take place, and further it may play a part in the aetiology of pain of vertebral origin; indeed, both seem quite likely. But the clinical assessment of bony position, together with the identification of the normal or abnormal state, is seen to be little more than a dream; and precisely the same arguments have to be applied to claims regarding the therapeutic repositioning of vertebrae. The clinician employing bony position diagnostically is clearly seen to be either ignorant of proven facts of substantial relevance, or choosing to ignore them. In either case, he must not be surprised that he is not accepted by an increasingly scientifically minded medical profession.

It was interesting that, of the participants in the workshop, two initially thought bony position to be of great importance, four of some importance and five of none. By the end of the workshop this had changed to three, four and five! Clearly, prior indoctrination has been effective.

15
Muscle function and its testing

Muscle function is a difficult and complex study. An enormous amount of work has been done in this field, much of it revealing serious deficiencies in earlier teaching[58]. Within musculoskeletal medicine, many beliefs are still held which do not take into consideration what is now known of the subject. Definitions of function of individual muscles to be found in standard textbooks of anatomy are often misleading[10]. The dedicated student of muscle function may find *Muscles Alive*[59] by Basmajian and DeLuca invaluable, but all physicians must be aware of certain facts in respect of muscle function, their control systems and the clinical testing of muscle strength. Perhaps most significant are the great sophistication of muscle function (including the variable manner in which recruitment and derecruitment of individual motor units takes place) and the complexity and unpredictability of the relevant control systems.

Of particular importance is that the control strategies for large and small muscles differ significantly, which is not surprising when one considers the very different functions of, for example, the erector spinae and the extrinsic muscles of the eye[59].

With regard to spinal muscle function, many orthodox ideas have been shown to be erroneous; in *Musculoskeletal Medicine, the Spine*[10], 30 items are listed in respect of the erector spinae, which demonstrates the inaccuracy and inadequacy of such an authority as *Gray's Anatomy*; a further 13 items in respect of the deep spinal muscles, and another 18 in respect of the abdominal muscles have been shown to play a part in this connection. For example, it may surprise some to learn that the erector spinae are at their most active in voluntary *flexion* of the spine[10]!

The importance of these considerations lies in what the relatively recent advances in knowledge mean to the clinician. The two chief areas of interest are muscle training and muscle strength testing.

Muscle training

The concept that a muscle's strength is increased by training is well established; but, sadly, while it is a very attractive idea, it is not entirely sound. What actually happens is that its efficiency is enhanced: the efficiency of the overall recruitment of its constituent motor units, and the efficiency of its interaction with antagonists and synergists[10]. The intrinsic strength of its individual fibres and groups of fibres is a totally different matter. And the fact remains that the effective strength of any muscle is in part a function of the perpendicular distance of its insertion from its fulcrum of movement. Clearly, these matters must all have an influence on how we teach exercises, as well as on how we assess muscle strength. While this question is outside the scope of this book, it should be borne in mind by all those involved in musculoskeletal medicine.

Muscle strength testing

This is not included in the basic system of case analysis that Burn and I have evolved for five cogent reasons:

1. The complexity of muscle action and interaction is such as to make meaningful clinical testing of strength of individual muscles virtually impossible[59].

2. Clinical methods of testing muscle strength are of necessity crude and non-specific. Literally dozens of muscles are in play in every instance of so-called individual muscle testing.

3. With regard to the traditional neurological examination, Magora et al. (1974)[60] examined 57 patients with headache syndromes and found EMG evidence of neuropathic or spinal lesions in the semispinalis muscles in a high proportion of them.

   Their second remarkable observation was the high incidence of neuropathic lesions disclosed by EMG, *even though a careful neurological examination had not revealed any pathological signs*[60]. Reliance upon the latter form of clinical assessment must therefore at best provide a relatively insensitive audit.

4. "Manual muscle tests are currently the primary procedure for determining muscular strength and the progression or regression of strength. Yet these tests are subjective, and their accuracy depends on the training, skill and experience of the clinician performing the examination. A relatively recent report stated that there are no quantitative methods for measuring muscle function in clinical use today . . . ."[59].

5. To quote Professor John Basmajian further, "When a muscle or group of muscles is weakened, there is a tendency for subtle shifts in the pattern of muscle activity to occur, to enable the synergistic muscles to generate the required force. This is known as muscle substitution, and it denies the impaired muscle the intended exercise"[59].

Clearly, this last is of fundamental importance: the phenomenon of muscle substitution can only mean that clinical muscle strength testing is of dubious diagnostic value; the examiner is gaining no more than a subjective impression of strength of a muscle or group which (because of muscle substitution) he cannot accurately identify. How strong does what feel?! There is no clinical way in which he can know which muscle, or muscles, he is testing!

While there is nothing to stop him using tests of muscle strength (if he finds them helpful), the clinician who continues to practise and teach them, without having shown these considerations to be wrong, cannot expect the approbation of his more scientifically minded colleagues – to be frank, neither will he deserve it.

16
Biomechanics in clinical practice

The experimental techniques for precise, no-risk, in vivo measurements in the human are yet to be developed.[55]

This statement is derived from none other than White and Panjabi, from which source the next five quotations are also drawn. What it means for the clinician is that the whole field is of almost exclusively academic interest and that it is unwise to lean very heavily upon biomechanics in the real life of the clinician.

The physiological muscle forces (applicable to the mobile segment) have not been simulated.[55]

In this case, is it acceptable in logic for us to interpret such experimental findings as there are as being valid in vivo? In view of the work of Basmajian and DeLuca[59], demonstrating the connectivity and plasticity of the neurological control of muscle function, thereby illustrating its resultant complete unpredictability, it seems that to do so would mean we were on very difficult ground indeed.

The characteristics of the force vectors that cause in vivo physiological motion are not known.[55]

If we do not know what is pulling in which direction and how hard, or what other forces are concurrently being applied to other related structures, what justification can there be for suggesting that we understand the biomechanics of human motion? If we look again at the evidence put forward by Basmajian and DeLuca, it is clearly impossible to determine clinically at any time what forces are being developed by which muscles in which direction.

Studies are done to simulate vertebral motion, but it is not known whether the motion experimentally produced is the same as that which is physiologically produced in vivo.[55]

If this is true, we have no right to assert that the results of such experimental work reflect the physiological truth. They *may* do so, but *we do not know* that they do. This is currently beyond proof.

The vectors that should represent the existing physiological preloads are not known.[55]

It follows that, just as we do not know the way the muscles work to produce movement, neither do we know how they work to maintain posture prior to that movement, or following it, nor how the constantly changing relationship between agonist, antagonist and synergist are governed.

At present we are not aware of published studies of kinematics that take [these matters] into consideration.[55]

The only sound interpretation of these six statements, quoted from acknowledged leading exponents in the field, is that, so far as it concerns vertebral joint movement, biomechanics remains an academic study of interest to some, at the same time having *no proven relevance to the clinician*. It is therefore not currently acceptable to make use of biomechanics to explain what we are doing, any more than it is to do so to justify our choice of therapy. Further, it can have *no diagnostic value*.

Two further matters are crucial to a sober assessment of biomechanics for the musculoskeletal physician. First, as with so many aspects of the human organism, there is almost certainly significant variation to be found in the precise points of insertion of muscles; if this were not the case, and if perfect symmetry were the rule, it would surely be an anatomical rarity! This is of importance as the effectiveness of muscle contraction is directly proportional to the distance of its insertion from the fulcrum of any resultant movement (if there is a fixed fulcrum!). For a fixed load, the moment of rotation depends upon the linear distance of its application from the fulcrum, perpendicular to the line of pull. And, of course, in vivo, often the fulcrum moves too, particularly in spinal movement.

Second, while it may be reasonable to consider biomechanics further with respect to peripheral joint movement, the spinal joints present a wholly different problem; not only can no spinal joint move in isolation (without breaking bone), no spinal segment can move relative to its immediate neighbours without moving them also. Whole regions of the spine move in unpredictable fashion, not only with respect to their numerous joints, but in a pattern determined by their equally unpredictable neuromuscular control mechancisms.

If the known unpredictability of the muscle control mechanisms and the proven phenomenon of muscle substitution determine that the strength of linear pull exerted by a muscle is unknown, and if this pull is delivered at an unknown distance from the fulcrum of rotation of the joint in question, so altering its effective moment, what is the point of talking about it to clinicians? I submit that the whole subject is restricted to an academic study, as least until such time as all White and Panjabi's clearly stated problems are resolved.

This is not to say that biomechanics is 'wrong', only to stress that its relevance to the clinician with respect to the spine is *very limited*, and that this must remain the case until these points are answered. In the mean time, for the clinician, it is no more than a very complex fantasy, even when it is adorned by two-dimensional illustrations of great sophistication.

I do not wish to be misquoted on this; biomechanics has already made substantial strides in the elucidation of a number of other matters of importance to the clinician. Perhaps of greatest importance, it has shown clearly the way in which destruction of transverse or vertical trabeculae affects the strength of cancellous bone under compression, and this in differing degree, due to the minute architecture of the bone. Loss of transverse trabeculae is very much less serious than that of vertical trabeculae, although the causative process may be precisely the same. This is of obvious importance in understanding osteoporosis, as also in the understanding of bony neoplasm. And, of course, in the manufacture of 'custom-built' prostheses, biomechanics plays a crucial part. But the experimental data relating to stresses and loads sufficient to overload the vertebral body, while they make fascinating reading as an independent study, are not yet of such validity as to be of consequence to the musculoskeletal clinician.

Of course, it is tempting to assume significance in being able to recite measurement figures – to describe movements in a jargon that sounds superficially scientific. But we have to look further than this if we are to be accepted as serious clinicians within orthodox medicine. We have to justify what we say in terms that all will understand.

I end by once more quoting Professor Panjabi, this time in person. At the end of his lecture on the subject to the 8th Congress of FIMM in 1986[61], he said, "I cannot see the relevance of this material to the work you do".

17
What of the intervertebral disc?
A second look

History

Sciatica was described by ancient Greek and Roman physicians. However, it was not until 1764 that it was first attributed to the sciatic nerve; much later it was attributed to spinal arthritis. Only in 1932 was it first attributed to disc protrusion[62]. Unhappily, little truly scientific work has since been directed to establishing the precise relationship between the disc and sciatic pain.

Currently, the disc is incriminated by different authors in from 95% to 5% of cases; such disparity in teaching must indicate an element of doubt! For this reason alone, too much conviction in this matter must raise the suspicions of the orthodox. We need valid evidence.

Anatomy

Functionally, the cartilaginous plates may be regarded as parts of the disc. The nucleus pulposus is well known to the whole profession, as are the annulus fibrosus, and the supporting ligaments lashing it into place.

The blood supply to each part is again well known, but there remains endless argument about innervation of the annulae. Once more, this seems to be a largely academic matter, rather than having any appreciable clinical significance, as the annulus and its supporting ligaments are in the closest apposition, so that any distortion of one demands a similar degree of distortion of the other, which means that potentially painful movements or strains are more or less equally shared. And, of course, innervation of the ligaments is well documented and undisputed[34].

Function

The disc is often said to be a load-bearing structure; although true on a part-time basis, this is NOT primarily so, as the early mammals originally stood and walked with their spines at about 45°, involving totally different stresses[22]. Over a long period, most mammals changed their dominant posture for a more or less horizontal one (with their own attendant problems) while man assumed the *part-time* erect posture. Even so, man's discs are indeed vertically load-bearing for only a surprisingly small part of his day.

Functionally, the disc allows modest mobility in flexion/extension, sidebending, rotation and shear, and limitless combinations of these. This permits adequate flexibility of the spine, coupled with considerable strength. To employ a simple engineering analogy, the disc forms a slightly mobile universal joint, almost incidentally able to take some compression load, due to the elasticity of the annulus and the deformability of the nucleus. As both the latter attributes are variable, both between individuals and within an individual over a period of time, it is not surprising that wide differences are observed, an unpredictable proportion of which may contribute to dysfunction.

Dysfunction

Degeneration (or ageing), inevitably involves a reduction in elasticity of the annulus and its supporting ligaments, as well as in deformability of the nucleus; accompanying osteophyte formation may accentuate the effects of these features by mechanically restricting joint range.

Excessive stresses, either prolonged of lesser degree or briefer of greater degree (or both) may give rise to bulging or rupture of the annulus, with inevitable damage to the associated ligament, perhaps accompanied by protrusion of nuclear material (amongst other things!). It is interesting that chondrocytes have been reported as the predominant cells found in excised disc material[63]. It is very important to remember that proven disc protrusions occur in 37% of pain-free subjects[64]. All scanning techniques may thereby prove clinically misleading, and the better the picture of a possibly innocent bulge, the more likely this seems to be. It is too easy to assume that a demonstrable bulge is clinically significant. Unnecessary surgery may result from this assumption, with little likelihood of a satisfactory result. It is reasonable to suggest that this may be a factor in determining the disappointing overall results of disc surgery.

Weakening of the supporting ligaments permits excessive movement, at times contributing to spondylolisthesis. Again, this is commonly asymptomatic[65]. Its demonstration may, therefore, also be misleading.

Ankylosing spondylitis reduces movement by inflammatory changes affecting in particular the ligaments.

Other pathology will not be dealt with here as it is unnecessary in a text for basic musculoskeletal teaching (but see Chapter 8).

In addition to pain, neurological manifestations of disc protrusion include muscle weakness, changes in reflexes and sensory changes. As already discussed in Chapter 15, there is a particular difficulty in the clinical estimation of weakness, chiefly as a result of the phenomenon of muscle substitution (which renders it clinically impossible to test a specific muscle). And it must be remembered that conditions other than disc protrusion may affect tendon reflexes, making their estimation a less clear test than most of us were taught. However, the importance of saddle anaesthesia and difficulties in micturition must be stressed, as these demand instant referral for urgent surgery[10].

Therapy

Therapies for the disc include analgesics, rest, heat, cold, massage, manipulation, traction, chemonucleolysis, acupuncture, TNS, etc., etc., ending with various forms of surgery. As mentioned above, the difficulties in assessment are illustrated by the surprisingly poor results of surgery[66]. These have little to do with the skill of the surgeon, rather stressing that removal of tissue *not* the cause of the clinical problem is unlikely to prove curative! There must be some significance in the great variety of therapies currently in use for problems still thought by some to arise predominantly in the disc.

Discussion in the workshop was revealing, in that, amongst an international group of teachers, an appreciable number were initially unaware of some of the facts outlined above.

18
What of the pelvis?

Much current teaching on this subject is based on unvalidated statements; this is a practice which seriously reduces the likelihood of acceptance of musculoskeletal medicine by serious members of the orthodox medical profession.

It is wise to commence with the known facts:

1. The bones of the pelvis, like the vertebrae rostral to them, are commonly NOT symmetrical; asymmetry is the rule, rather than the exception[10].

2. The sacroiliac joints, perhaps too often incriminated as a source of pain, are of considerable surface area, grossly irregular in contour, normally asymmetrical in the individual, and bound very firmly together anteriorly and posteriorly by the ligaments, thus allowing VERY little movement. Apart from the interosseous sutures of the cranium, this must be the nearest approach to joint 'locking' to be found – and it is, of course, wholly physiological.

3. The symphysis pubis is also a VERY strong joint, cushioned by its disc and supported by thick tough ligaments on all sides. Like the sacroiliac joints, it is designed to move VERY little, permitting minimal realignment in all directions; again the main function of this disc is NOT load bearing between its two facets, but rather that of permitting a *very* small degree of most movements. It is a shock-absorber.

4. The sacrococcygeal joint is rather less robustly built, but it is reasonable to suggest that this is related to the fact that it is normally subjected to relatively minor stresses. This is reflected in the fact that the anterior and posterior ligaments are not so massive as those mentioned so far.

5. The hip joints are, of course, a part of the pelvis, but these are not to be discussed now, except to mention that they are subject to great stresses and repeated shocks. This is reflected in their system of very strong ligaments, and also in their liability to degeneration.

6. Like the intervertebral joints, the pelvic joints are subject to degenerative changes; also they are at times the site of inflammatory changes, such as sacroiliitis – both demonstrable at some stage on various types of scanning.

7. The ligaments holding the pelvic basin together are arguably the strongest in the entire body. For this reason, they must be LESS likely to suffer strain; even the bony parts are 'stayed' by the inguinal ligaments.

8. Because of the common incidence of the twin phenomena of referred pain and referred tenderness, it is difficult to demonstrate with any certainty a local origin for pain perceived over these joints. For example, sacroiliac pain may frequently be shown to be referred from the thoracolumbar spine; pain from this region may also be referred to other parts of the pelvis (including the hip)[47]. Equally important, superficial fibres of the dorsal branches of L1 and L2 have been traced over the iliac crest, to directly innervate the upper buttock[45].

In view of these facts, quite apart from the subjectivity involved in the search for signs, complex biomechanical explanations of supposed pelvic movement, as are currently commonly taught, must remain hypothetical, as must the inference that such small-amplitude articular shifts are common causes of pain and disability. Of course there is movement in all these joints, but it is small in range, complex, always in conjunction with other joint movements and of little proven importance to the clinician.

In the same way, detailed descriptions of therapeutic procedures based on such hypotheses remain unvalidated; in practice such manoeuvres are far from specific. To be persuaded of this, one has but to watch a so-called 'specific' manipulation of, say, the sacroiliac joint; very many structures are involved in a great non-specific upheaval! From a practical point of view, in the present state of knowledge, such theories as these can have little clinical significance, and, unhappily, they serve to reduce the likelihood of acceptance of musculoskeletal medicine by the (very properly) scientifically critical.

19
Posture put in its place

Three definitions of posture warrant consideration.

1. "The position the body assumes in preparation for the next movement."[67] This definition implies intent, which cannot be justifiable in a definition of a static concept; posture must surely have an independent existence.

2. "Standing on one leg."[68] This definition, though widely used within musculoskeletal medicine, is really more an illustration of a part of posture. Of course, standing on one leg brings into play a whole range of posturally related functions, in themselves of more than passing academic interest, and a change of leg results in complex widespread neuromuscular and articular adjustments. However, it is clear that it defines nothing and so has, regrettably, little sound scientific basis in this sense.

3. "Short-term or long-term arrest of those neuromuscular changes which determine both articular and non-articular movement." In effect, it is 'putting on hold' a whole range of complex neuromuscular activities; it may be thought of as a single frame in a cine-film of movement. (I offer this as my personal definition.)

It is difficult to determine the clinical significance of posture. Indeed, its intrinsic significance (other than aesthetic, or as a part of communication) has never been clearly shown. It *may* have a dual role in pathogenesis and prophylaxis but this remains a hypothetical consideration, in spite of what is widely taught on the subject.

The structures which may be affected are several, and are perhaps best considered in groups.

1. Quite apart from the train of neurological activity induced by distorting these structures, the joint capsules and their supporting ligaments may be subjected to prolonged stress. The resultant stretching may prove irreversible if continued too long, although recovery from short-term stretching is usually rapid and complete.

2. While the muscles and tendons are the obvious chief mediators of both maintenance and change in posture, they may themselves suffer from prolonged over-use.

3. Blood vessels are relatively seldom considered in a postural context, but it is clear that arterial flow may be impaired by protracted kinking or compression due to postural factors.

Venous stasis can arise from the same cause or from the withdrawal of the physiological 'muscle pump' associated with frequent changes in posture which are the essence of movement.

4. Nerve roots may similarly be affected by posture. Minimal compression or traction may have no harmful effects in the short term, but, maintained for long periods, they may result in changes sufficient to produce symptoms. Such changes may prove irreversible.

Posture may act as a pathogen in more than one way. Extremes of movement imposing acute strains on any of the structures mentioned may prove pathogenic. The prolonged maintenance of chronic strains on the same structures may also prove pathogenic.

However, it is difficult to incriminate any particular postural factors with any certainty in view of the wide variation of conformation of individuals and the unpredictability of function of the nervous system, coupled with the fact that it is seldom that any one factor presents on its own.

Posture is often acclaimed as important in prophylaxis. While it is clear that the avoidance of the extremes of movement, and of movement that is too rapid and uncontrolled, seems sensible, there is as yet insufficient evidence to validate this view to the satisfaction of the sceptical.

Similarly, it is reasonable to suggest that improvement of the possible range of movement by gentle stretching exercises may reduce the likelihood of over-reaching the 'normal' range for the individual.

Again, avoidance of certain specific chronic stresses seems reasonable. Posture at work has been the subject of much study. This has included standing, sitting and working in awkward positions, repetitive tasks and vibration, but, unhappily, the study of ergonomics has to date contributed little to our understanding of the role of posture. The chief difficulty lies in isolating particular features[69]. Nearly always multiple factors are at work, making the incrimination of any one cause extremely difficult.

Posture while travelling has also been widely studied. Standing, sitting and lying each has its own problems, as again has vibration. Car seat design has been the object of enormous research expenditure, although less thought has been given to teaching the driver to keep his bottom in the desired place! All these factors *may* be of relevance but none is clearly of prime importance.

Posture relaxing at home presents further problems. Of course, sitting may be a source of trouble for the back, but, again, there is little sound evidence in this field. Once more, both the clinician and the potential patient need to remain empiricists.

Bed is perhaps the most dangerous place of all! Enormous sums of money have been wasted in the purchase of special beds. Until the sleeper has learned to sleep in a particular part of the bed, in a particular posture, and to stay there all night, it seems unlikely that a posturally satisfactory bed will emerge unless the bed is designed to automatically change its physical characteristics with changes of posture. The only such bed of which I am aware failed to attract a manufacturer! And further, of course, we remain uncertain of the inherent disadvantages of protracted non-movement; this may itself prove pathogenic. Perhaps an uncomfortable bed is at times an advantage!

Congenital variations in form are often assumed to be causative of back problems. As with the normal signs of degeneration and bony asymmetry, this is commonly NOT the case: the body usually compensates well.

In view of the above, it seems clear that too-great certainty in the matter of posture is likely to produce as many problems as it solves! It is highly significant that the word 'may' occurs sixteen times in this chapter so far. The lesson to be learned from this is that we must be strongly suspicious of teaching in this subject which is too assured. The truth is – we do not know!

With respect to gait, there exist a number of beliefs involving the ability to make diagnostic predictions on the slender evidence of watching a patient walk across a room. In view of the number of variables connected with posture (inevitably the more complex on assuming movement), it seems likely that these beliefs will remain unproven. It is perhaps significant that gait, like posture, is affected by many factors, including those which are anatomical, physiological, pathological, emotional and contrived. In the field of rehabilitation, of course, gait may be very important, particularly in monitoring progress. But its diagnostic importance must be carefully weighed in view of the evidence now available.

In spite of these factors, eight of the participants in the workshop commenced with the belief that posture and gait were of great diagnostic importance in musculoskeletal medicine, three regarding them as of some importance. Surprisingly, these figures altered only slightly over the four days, ending with seven attaching great importance to them, three some and two none.

20
The future of musculoskeletal medicine

Judging by the relatively few reviews which have been made in recent years, and without those adjustments which are seen to be required in both undergraduate and postgraduate teaching as indicated earlier in this book, the academic standing of musculoskeletal medicine still seems to be somewhat unsatisfactory in many countries. Indeed, with a few important exceptions, there is currently something of a shadow over the question of its acceptance by the orthodox establishment. Nonetheless, in a number of countries, there are those who believe that it should now be regarded as a medical speciality in its own right. There are four crucial factors which need to be considered before coming to an informed judgement as to the validity of this view and as to what influence such an attitude may have on the future of musculoskeletal medicine.

1. Musculoskeletal medicine in fact spreads throughout the whole spectrum of clinical practice; this can only mean that it should be taught at a basic level to all clinicians, rather than as a special subject to relatively few enthusiasts. Before this can happen, it must be accepted as a legitimate part of orthodox medicine.

2. Justification of any claim for musculoskeletal medicine to be on an academic par with, for example, orthopaedic surgery or rheumatology, requires very much more than the relatively brief postgraduate training programmes which have been proposed in certain quarters. Such a suggestion could readily be taken as an affront to those of established specialist/consultant status, a sort of snollygoster's charter*. Indeed, to prove acceptable, this sort of development would demand of the candidate proper, long-term work under supervision, as well as accreditation to a standard which meets the highest academic demands. (See Chapter 1.)

3. Those who choose to take the peculiar interests and therapies of musculoskeletal medicine further may readily do so with the postgraduate facilities currently available, but, because of the unavoidable empiricism obtaining in this field, coupled with the unpredictability of therapeutic

---

*Snollygoster: a burgeoning politician with no platform, principles, or party preference[70]

outcome, they will still from time to time need to refer patients to existing specialists, in particular to rheumatologists, orthopaedic and neurosurgeons, neurologists or pain clinics, as the occasion demands.

4. More important, advocates of immediate specialist status are unlikely to gain the wholehearted support of those specialists upon whom they must clinically continue to depend, appearing to be in competition, rather than as therapeutically complementary.

These four factors present a strong argument in favour of better undergraduate teaching in this field, coupled with opportunities for postgraduate study largely for general practitioners (who, after all, in most countries are likely to continue to see the majority of these patients). A further factor confusing the issue is that the word 'specialist' has different connotations in different countries; it should not be confused with the word 'consultant'. It seems unlikely that undergraduate teaching will be widely adjusted before the postgraduate scene has been clarified and basic musculoskeletal medicine has become legitimate. The latter is the realistic, if limited, long-term goal of this book.

Much of the postgraduate training necessary for this purpose is peculiarly well suited to distance package learning, so ably shown in the United Kingdom by the Open University and others to be highly effective. While assumed by some to be inferior to older established methods of teaching, in fact, this system offers more individual tuition rather than less and is far better suited to the needs of the busy practitioner! It also promotes a greater degree of standardization of both syllabus and teaching method. Those parts of such an educational programme as are not amenable to this discipline are already available in several countries, and international co-ordination of basic syllabi and teaching practices would seem a natural development of considerable potential. Indeed, this was the reason the Fédération Internationale de Médecine Manuelle recently promoted the workshop for teachers from twelve different countries, and the further workshop to be held in 1995: in an attempt to reach consensus in basic teaching.

Such an approach is particularly appropriate to general practice; it is also readily realizable. In the United Kingdom, respectability of musculoskeletal medicine has now been achieved, under the auspices of the University of Bath and with the co-ordination of the Primary Care Rheumatology Society, as an integral part of that University's Postgraduate Diploma in Primary Care Rheumatology. This represents wholehearted academic acceptance – an orthodox status for musculoskeletal medicine and the recognition of vertebral manipulation as a scientifically acceptable therapeutic option, rather than a system of complementary medicine. Broadly comparable acceptance has also been won in some other countries (particularly in France) although the syllabus is not yet widely standardized internationally.

In the United Kingdom, a further factor is of fundamental importance. The Department of Health clearly recognizes both the nature and the proportions of the problem of musculoskeletal medicine (and particularly that of back pain) and it is currently actively pursuing a policy directed towards ensuring these problems *are dealt with very largely in general practice*. The Provident Associations share this appreciation. Enormous financial savings for both are likely to accrue from the adoption of this policy (see First Foreword).

The financial advantages will also become apparent in general practice, where suitably qualified doctors will enable practices to save substantially on both drugs and referrals, simply by treating patients in this field themselves. The new Postgraduate Diploma in Primary Care Rheumatology will help to identify general practitioners competent to play this role. Judging by the response to the recent international teachers' workshop, the scene appears to be set for other countries to follow suit. Indeed, the possibility of a European postgraduate diploma in musculoskeletal medicine is currently under discussion. It is but a short and logical step from this welcome postgraduate advance to the inclusion of musculoskeletal medicine in the orthodox undergraduate curriculum – by invitation, rather than by confrontational demand.

On this basis, I see a solid increase in safe down-to-earth vertebral manipulation within general practice as being very likely indeed; in this view, I am joined by a substantial number of very senior members of the medical profession. It appears that this trend may well prove to be international; to the considerable benefit of patients. In view of the proportions of the problem, this is a change which I see as being urgent.

However, without the benefit of a recognizable and recognized basic platform, such as is now emerging, the demands that have been made worldwide by a variety of enthusiasts over the past fifty years have not been met with widespread success; perhaps we should all learn from this fact. Frankly, there seems to be little sound scientific support for similar proposals at the present time. This statement does not infer that I am opposed to specialist status for musculoskeletal physicians; far from it, although on a number of occasions I have voiced my concern over the manner in which this may best be achieved.

Of course, there is an understandable attraction in being professionally 'up-graded' but this is surely of far less urgency than the encouragement of doctors to look critically at what has been taught in the past and to observe the significant, if overdue, changes which are currently taking place in this field. As it see it, once acceptance of musculoskeletal medicine is more widely established on a no-nonsense physiological basis, it would not be altogether surprising for a speciality to emege – as a convenience for the medical profession rather than as something demanded by yet another group of enthusiasts. First, we need acceptance of the basics.

Appendix 1
Participants in first FIMM teachers' workshop – Vienna, 1994

In the enforced absence of Professor Joan Garcia-Alsina and Dr Loïc Burn, the workshop was presented by Dr John Paterson, La Roque D'Antheron, France.
The following participated in the workshop:

Dr Guido Brugnoni, Italy
Dr Gabor Ormos, Hungary
Dr Peter Gabriel, Belgium
Dr Marc-Henri Gauchat, Switzerland
Dr Markus Hanna, Austria
Dr Jean-Yves Maigne, France
Dr Jukka Mannevaara, Finland
Dr Annett Ockhuysen, Holland
Dr Glen Gorm Rasmussen, Denmark
Dr Lars-Erik Strender, Sweden
Dr John Tanner, United Kingdom
Dr Johannes Weingart, Germany

I wish to express my sincere gratitude to all those participating in the workshop, without whose enthusiasm this book could not have been completed. I look forward to real progress in the second workshop.

Appendix 2
Analysis of initial workshop questionnaires

Age group

31–40	1
41–50	8
51–60	2

Occupation

General practitioners	2

Specialists	
Manual medicine	1
Rheumatology	3
Orthopaedic	1
Sports medicine	1
Rehabilitation	2
Internist	1
Total	9

Countries represented

Austria	Holland
Belgium	Hungary
Denmark	Italy
Finland	Sweden
France	Switzerland
Germany	United Kingdom

One participant from each country.

Position in association

President	2
Secretary	2
Treasurer	1
Regular teacher	11

Questions

		Certainly	*Perhaps*	*No*
1.	Do you think co-ordination of *basic* teaching within FIMM is desirable?	10	1	0
2.	Do you think co-ordination of *basic* teaching within FIMM is possible?	3	8	0

		Great	*Some*	*None*
3.	How much diagnostic importance do you attach to the following?			
a.	Joint mobility	9	1	1
b.	Bony position	2	4	5
c.	Muscle strength testing	3	7	1
d.	Clinical biomechanics	7	4	0
e.	Radiology, etc.	5	5	0
f.	Posture and gait	8	3	0
g.	Pelvic movements and alignment	4	6	0

		Yes	*No*
4.	Are the following subjects currently taught in your association's basic courses?		
a.	Epidemiology of back pain (supporting text used . . . Tilscher)	5	5
b.	Pain perception and modulation (supporting text used . . . Zimmermann)	9	2
c.	Referred pain and tenderness (supporting text used . . . Brugger)	11	0
d.	Relevant anatomy (supporting text used . . . Fick Benninghof)	11	0
e.	Relevant pathology (supporting text used . . . Tilscher)	10	1

Comments

The twelve particpants represented a broad cross-section of the Fédération Internationale de Médecine Manuelle with a high proportion of them in the 41–50 age group. All were regular teachers in their respective countries, and five of them held office in their national associations. Almost all were convinced that international co-ordination of basic teaching was desirable, though only three really expected success in this endeavour.

The remaining figures confirm the impression gained from the survey of teaching referred to in the text[5], that variations in presentation and syllabus between member associations are wide. They also indicate to some extent the direction of bias from the orthodox commonly found. Comment on individual items is to be found in the appropriate chapters, or will be made in the comparison in Appendix 3.

Appendix 3
Analysis of final workshop questionnaire

	Yes	No
1. Has the workshop changed your general approach to the teaching of *basic* musculoskeletal medicine?	2	10

If yes, in what way?   No reasons offered

2. How much diagnostic importance do you now attach to the following?

	Great	Some	None
a. Joint mobility	9 (9)*	1 (1)†	1 (1)
b. Bony position	3 (2)	4 (4)	5 (5)
c. Muscle strength testing	1 (3)	10 (7)	1 (1)
d. Clinical biomechanics	6 (7)	5 (4)	1 (0)
e. Radiology, etc.	1 (5)	11 (5)	0 (0)
f. Posture and gait	7 (8)	3 (3)	2 (0)
g. Pelvic movements and alignment	6 (4)	6 (6)	0 (0)

3. Are there any deletions you would like to recommend from the current *basic* syllabus of your country?   Less theory

4. Are there any additions you would like to make to the current *basic* syllabus of your country?

            More epidemiology
                More practicals
       Different manual techniques

---

*Numbers in parentheses are the results of the initial questionnaires
†One marked a reply between some and none!

	Yes	*No*
5. What help do you think FIMM could/should offer in making the changes you think desirable?		
a. Further workshop(s) for teachers	10**	1
b. Basic international courses for beginners	4	8
c. Is there any further assistance you would welcome from FIMM?		

Develop European education standard in MM	1
Promotion of work for physicians educated in FIMM	1
Help in translations for submission of papers	1
Information/recommendation for education	1
Educational programmes from other countries	1
Criteria for diploma in MM	2
Better communication within FIMM	1
Develop 'gold standard' for basic teaching	1
Develop 'gold standard' for specialist training	1
Acceptance of proposed analysis sheet	1
Basic syllabus	2
Time schedule for other countries	1
Data bank in scientific teaching	1
Report concerning EEC integration	1

6. If you answered 'yes' to 5a, which options would you favour?

1995	7
Later	4
On-going series (at what frequency?)	
annually	1
biennially	1
triennially	1
Vienna again	5
Another venue (please suggest one)	5
Amsterdam	2
France	1
Zurich	1
Paris	1

**The goal of any future meeting should be more specific. Such a meeting should be integrated with a FIMM meeting

	Yes	No
7. If you answered 'yes' to 5b, should this include further material?		

	Yes	No
a. Injections	1	2
b. Drugs	0	2
c. Collars, corsets, traction and bedrest	1	2
d. Other (please suggest topics)		
Neuromuscular	1	1

Comment: It is important to differentiate musculoskeletal medicine from chiropractic and osteopathy.

	Yes	No
8. Do you think the basic non-sectarian approach found in the workshop will help in gaining acceptance of musculoskeletal medicine within orthodoxy in your country?	9 (1)	2

Comments:
FIMM should formulate general recommendations for a diploma in Europe.
Some countries already regard musculoskeletal medicine as orthodox.

Assessment

The first comment must be to note the degree to which participants changed their minds: in general terms, as revealed by the answers to question 1, and in specific areas, as revealed in question 2. This is the result of discussing relevant matters in the light of a common scientific base. I find the small degree of change quite extraordinary, and it reveals a level of indoctrination sufficient to annul an inherent wish to be regarded as members of the orthodox medical profession, rather than as being in some way complementary.

This interpretation is reinforced by the answers to questions 3 and 4, where a rather vague inclination is translated into something of a directive. But it is an area where FIMM may be able to offer some help, as indicated in the answers to questions 5–8. In particular, a 9:2 vote of confidence in a non-sectarian approach to gaining acceptance within orthodoxy is perhaps the most encouraging result of the 1994 workshop. It is likely that FIMM will deliberate seriously on these matters, and it will certainly be interesting to observe the response to this exercise. As a part of this process, it is hoped that this small book will prove helpful to all those who seek a scientifically acceptable base for musculoskeletal medicine.

Appendix 4
A basic musculoskeletal medicine syllabus

It is stressed that this syllabus is devised for international use, with emphasis on its scientific acceptability to the orthodox medical profession as a platform upon which to build. Based on that employed by myself and Loïc Burn since 1983, it has evolved over a number of years, more recently through discussion in the first teachers' workshop sponsored by FIMM. It aims to provide the novice with a scientifically sound basis for practice in this field, in safety and with reasonable expectation of therapeutic success. It is not intended to cater for specialist practice.

The importance of teaching being supported by texts which are themselves acceptable to the orthodox profession cannot be too strongly stressed. Regardless of their origins, orthodox or complementary, all hypotheses must be subjected to the same level of critical evaluation (a major aspect of the workshop). New and valid evidence must *always* demand reconsideration of current beliefs and teaching (see Chapter 1).

In accordance with this principle, the syllabus deliberately excludes items unacceptable to the orthodox medical profession. At the same time (as far as possible), it avoids the use of specific jargon. Some of these exclusions may be surprising. For this reason, a list of the major ones is given after the syllabus, with a brief indication of why they are currently not acceptable: *such unacceptability is equally applicable to those texts which include these items in a basic framework*.

Stripped down to the bare essentials, the syllabus necessarily includes items of relevance to an understanding of the field and its practice, stressing the importance of the practitioner frequently not having the benefit of a valid diagnosis. This exposes an inescapable empiricism, perfectly acceptable so long as he is aware of it, and so long as he admits it, both privately and publicly! Much of the basic scientific learning required may be achieved by reading – in the doctor's home and at his convenience (see Chapter 20).

The time necessary to teach each item has been discussed at length, the recommendations here being realistic figures based on the assumption that scientifically acceptable texts have been previously digested. This may be ascertained by suitable accreditation: the latter is widely agreed to be desirable and may be readily grafted onto this base. The pattern that Burn and I have adopted informally is practicable, at the same time being searching of the candidate's grasp of the subject. Assuming the candidate has first thoroughly mastered the written manual, it involves practical assessment by both tutors, the submission of four case histories, a multiple-choice paper of eighty questions and an essay paper of four questions. A base text is used[71].

Syllabus

Subject	Initial instruction	Revision
Epidemiology	Text	20 min
Pain perception and modulation	Text	20 min
Referred pain and tenderness	Text	20 min
Psychology of pain (including psychological therapies)	Text	20 min
Relevant anatomy	Text	20 min
Relevant pathology	Text	20 min
The intervertebral disc	Text	20 min
The pelvis	Text	20 min
Trigger points and tender points	Text	10 min
Common presentations	Text	30 min
Case analysis	Text	30 min
Local examination	Text	60 min
The place of radiology, etc.	Text	20 min
Indications and contraindications	Text	20 min
Twelve basic manipulative techniques	24 h	6 h
Appropriate injections (including caudal epidurals)	Text	60 min
Miscellaneous therapies	Text	30 min

It will be seen that it is possible to reduce drastically the amount of time taken in practical courses by the prior use of a suitable text. This must be thoroughly read prior to a student coming on a practical course. In this way, the above syllabus may be fitted into a series of three two-day courses; this has the added advantage of students being able to perform limited techniques between courses and to put their personal experience to good use in subsequent courses.

Exclusions

Joint mobility – because it is known to vary widely in the cadaver and in the asymptomatic, and without correlation with any particular factors. Normal range thus being clinically unidentifiable, it follows that abnormal range must remain so also. Of course, any assessment of the quality of movement remains wholly subjective.

Bony position – because it is known that bony form varies widely, both between individuals and from one segmental level to the next, asymmetry being the rule, so that the subjective estimation of differences in bony prominence does not indicate either normal or abnormal position.

Muscle strength testing – because of the known unpredictability of muscle control systems and the phenomenon of muscle substitution, coupled with the subjective nature of most clinical testing, the clinician is denied identification of the axial muscle under test.

Clinical biomechanics – because of the five factors cited by Professor Panjabi (see Chapter 16):

The experimental techniques for precise no-risk in-vivo measurements in the human are yet to be developed.

The physiological muscle forces (applicable to the mobile segment) have not been simulated.

The characteristics of the force vectors that cause in-vivo physiological motion are not known.

Vertebral motion is being studied but it is not known whether the motion produced is the same as that which is physiologically produced in vivo.

The vectors that should represent the existing physiological preloads are not known.

Posture and gait – because these studies are based on subjective impressions, they are clinically immeasurable, of necessity remaining hypothetical.

It is proposed that the wide use of such a skeleton syllabus for basic teaching would contribute to the acceptance of musculoskeletal medicine within the orthodox medical profession. Details will change with the demands of sound research but its basis must remain scientific. A core of a few countries adopting this syllabus for their elementary courses would further permit the useful exchange of teachers and international co-ordination within FIMM.

If desired, advanced teaching may be adapted appropriately, founded firmly on such an orthodox base, thereby gaining acceptance by the orthodox.

Appendix 5
Twelve manipulative techniques described

Introduction

The most important aspect of describing manipulative techniques is the avoidance of specific jargon. As will be seen, this is quite possible. Description based on a variety of ideas about what is being attempted or achieved is perhaps the most cogent reason for the widespread rejection of manipulation by the orthodox medical profession. Here, descriptions are based on the anatomy and physiology all will know and accept.

Illustrations have been deliberately kept to a minimum, offering no more than a crude insight into what is described. The reason for this is that, the better the presentation, the greater is the temptation for the novice to dispense with a practical mode of learning manipulative skills; this is a recipe for second-rate techniques, if not for disaster. Manipulative skills must be learned 'in the flesh', rather than as an academic exercise. There is no substitute for this.

Further, this book is written partly for experienced manipulators, some of whom may harbour ingrained preconceptions, and partly for total novices, who may well be initially sceptical.

Why choose these particular techniques? They have been chosen for three reasons:

1. They are relatively simple in execution, thus easy to teach and to learn.

2. They are sufficient to offer the novice a choice in each region of the spine, enabling him to make early use of vertebral manipulation in practice, *after a suitable practical course*.

3. They demonstrate to the medical profession at large that vertebral manipulation need not be regarded as a mystic rite of great complexity, but is rather *the practical and very unsophisticated exploitation of accepted physiological phenomena in the relief of pain*.

It is interesting that all practising manipulators in fact evolve their own personal techniques; this is usually achieved by the gradual modification (and perhaps slight sophistication) of the basic procedures they start with. Every technique is subsequently modified in relation to the size, conformation and current neuromuscular state of each individual patient. The essential is that the novice commences with a clear understanding of the basic principles involved, coupled with a competence in a few relatively simple techniques. While some manipulators are taught many techniques, most, in practice, employ only quite a small range of techniques on an every-day basis. The twelve basic techniques described here are those broadly agreed by the first international teachers' workshop of FIMM as being an acceptable starting point.

Cervical technique 1
Upper cervical rotation – supine

Positioning

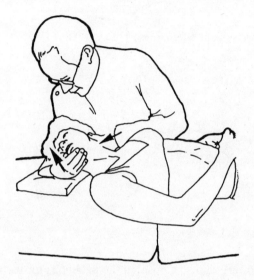

Adjust the couch level to your umbilicus: lie the patient supine, with her head supported in a position of comfort. Stand to the left of her head and, lying your right forearm beside her right ear, roll her head on to your forearm, your fingers just cupping her chin. Place the midshaft of the proximal phalanx of your left index finger over the left articular pillar at the level you wish to manipulate, your left thumb pointing anteriorly. To manipulate the upper segments, bend the neck over the fulcrum of your left index finger, and take up the slack in both right rotation and extension, maintaining close contact between the patient's head and your chest.

Manipulation

The final thrust is an accentuation of the positioning, your left index finger increasing extension by thrusting towards your right palm. This movement must be performed on a relaxed patient.

Cervical technique 2
Lower cervical rotation – supine

Positioning

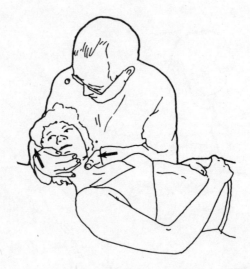

To manipulate the lower segments, position the patient as for the upper segments, rotating to the right, and extending the neck. Place the midshaft of the proximal phalanx of your left index finger over the left articular pillar at the level you wish to manipulate, your left thumb pointing anteriorly. Then bend the neck towards the patient's chest, over the fulcrum of your left index finger. Take up the slack, maintaining close contact between her head and your chest.

Manipulation

The final thrust is an accentuation of the positioning, as in the upper segment manoeuvre, again with your left index finger thrusting towards your right palm. The movement must be rapid and of short amplitude.

Cervical technique 3
Upper cervical rotation in traction – sitting

Positioning

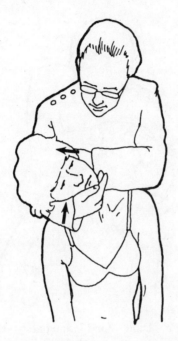

Seat the patient comfortably on a chair. Stand immediately behind the patient. Reaching over her right shoulder with your right arm, ask the patient to turn her head to the left and drop the right side of her head on to your right wrist. The fingers of your right hand cup her chin. Place the heel of your left hand over the patient's left occiput, the thumb along the occipital ridge, the fingers extending over the parietal bone.

Manipulation

Ensure the patient is relaxed, then take up the slack in left rotation, flexion and right side-bending, at the same time exerting quite a strong vertical traction with the right forearm, bringing her head into close contact with your chest. The final thrust is a rapid, short-amplitude accentuation of the positioning.

Cervical technique 4
Lower cervical rotation in extension – sitting

Positioning

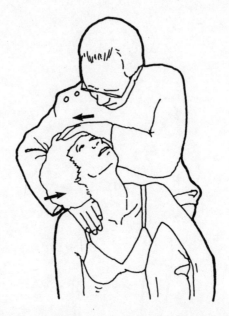

Seat the patient sideways on a chair. Stand immediately behind her and place your left foot on the seat of the chair, adjacent to her left hip. Drape the patient's left arm over your left thigh and apply your right thumb to the right side of her 7th cervical spinous process. Ask the patient to lean her head to the right and rotate left. Place your left palm on her left forehead and take up the slack in left rotation, extension and right side-bending, ensuring her head is closely applied to your chest.

Manipulation

The final thrust is a rapid, short-amplitude accentuation of the positioning. The patient must be relaxed at the moment of thrust.

Thoracic technique 1
Sternal thrust – standing

Positioning

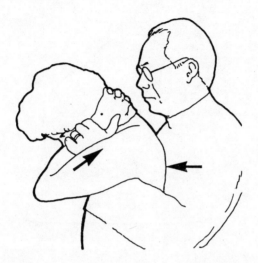

Ask the patient to stand relaxed. Standing behind her, ask her to link her fingers behind her neck, pass your forearms anterior to her upper arms, so as to clasp her wrists with your hands. Fold the patient's elbows forwards and flex her neck. Ask her to flex her neck, applying your sternum to her back, at the level you wish to manipulate. By flexing your arms at the elbow pull the patient towards your chest.

Manipulation

When the slack is taken up, apply a thrust rapidly and with restraint, by accentuation of the positioning, the thrust being applied by your sternum.

Positioning: a modification for tall patients

To position your sternum, ask the patient to keep her feet still and relax, reassure her that you will not drop her, and pull her over backwards, moving your feet back at the same time, until such time as the desired level of her thoracic spine is in contact with your sternum. You may find it 'safer' to move back against a wall or sturdy piece of furniture.

Thoracic technique 2
Sternal thrust – supine

Positioning

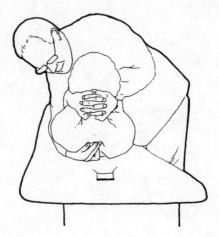

The patient lies supine, arms crossed. Stand to her right and, rolling her towards you, place your right thenar eminence over the left transverse process, your hand crossing the midline, all fingers being on the right of her spinous process of choice. Roll her back on to your right hand, clasping her elbows with your left hand, and flex her cervicothoracic spine to the required degree and apply your sternum closely over your left hand and her forearms.

Manipulation

Take up the slack, and make a rapid, short manipulative thrust with your sternum vertically towards your right thenar eminence.

Thoracic technique 3
Crossed pisiform thrust

Positioning

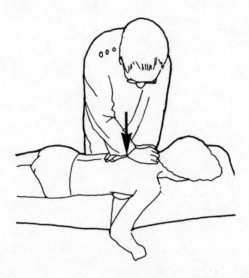

Lie the patient prone. Select the level at which manipulation is desired, remembering that the tips of the thoracic spinous processes overlap the vertebra below. Stand on the patient's left and place your left pisiform bone over her left 5th transverse process, the fingers and thumb pointing to your right. Place your right pisiform bone over her right 4th transverse process, the fingers and thumb pointing to your left.

Manipulation

Bending well over the patient, lean vertically downwards, both elbows slightly flexed, taking up the slack. Ask her to inhale deeply and then exhale. At the end of exhalation increase the downward force by a sharp, controlled thrust, achieved by extending both elbows simultaneously.

For the sake of description, this manoeuvre is part aimed at rotating the 4th thoracic vertebra anticlockwise on the 5th.

Thoracic technique 4
Thoracic rotation – sitting

Positioning

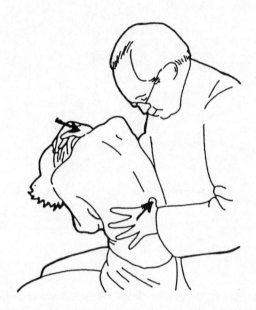

Adjust the couch level to just above your patellae. Sit the patient on the couch, legs apart, her hands clasped behind her neck. Pass your right hand anterior to her right upper arm and bring it to overlie her hands. Place your left thumb on the left lateral aspect of the spinous process at the level to be manipulated. Rotate her trunk to the right and bring her into marked flexion, leaning your chest on her right scapular region.

Manipulation

Taking up the slack, this is a rapid, short-amplitude thrust with your left thumb simultaneous to accentuation of rotation and flexion with your right arm and chest.

Lumbar technique 1
Lumbar rotation – supine

Positioning

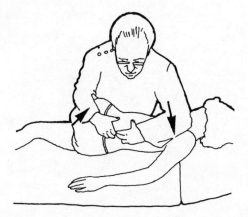

Lie the patient on her right side, her head lying on her right hand. Stand in front of her. Rotate her trunk to the left by placing your left forearm in the sulcus between her left shoulder and chest. Flex her left knee and hip, and place your right forearm over her left upper buttock. With fingers of both hands palpate the spinous processes above and below the level you wish to move. Use both forearms to increase rotation, monitoring the resultant movement with your finger tips.

Manipulation

Taking up the slack, the manipulation is executed by a sharp increase of rotatory pressure by both forearms, as illustrated.

This technique may be modified for higher levels by pulling her right shoulder forwards and downwards, thereby increasing thoracolumbar flexion.

Lumbar technique 2
Lumbar rotation – sitting

Positioning.

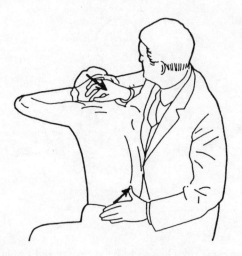

Adjust the couch level to just above your patellae. Sit the patient on the couch, legs apart, his hands clasped behind his neck. Pass your right hand anterior to his right upper arm and bring it to overlie his hands. Place your left thumb on the left lateral aspect of the spinous process at the level to be manipulated. Rotate his trunk to the right and bring him into flexion, leaning your chest on his right scapular area.

Manipulation

Taking up the slack, this is a rapid, short-amplitude thrust with your left thumb simultaneous to accentuation of rotation and flexion with your right arm and chest.

Lumbar technique 3
Lumbosacral thrust – prone

Positioning

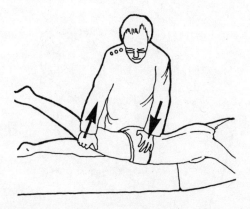

Lie the patient prone. Stand on the patient's left side (for a right-sided problem). Place the heel of your left hand over her right sacroiliac joint, bearing down firmly. With your right hand grasp the anterior aspect of her right thigh, just above the knee, hyperextending her right hip, taking up the slack.

Manipulation

Thrust vertically downwards with your left hand, while accentuating hyperextension of her right hip with your right hand.

Lumbar technique 4
Lumbosacral sagittal thrust

Positioning

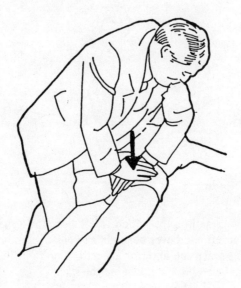

Adjust couch level to just above your patellae. Lie the patient on his right side at the edge of the couch, his left leg hanging over the edge of the couch. Grasp his left leg between your thighs, so as to provide stability. Place the heel of either hand over his left posterior superior iliac spine, reinforcing the downward pressure with your other hand.

Manipulation

This is a rapid, short-amplitude vertical thrust.

It is stressed that this selection of techniques has been arrived at after discussion within a group of experienced medical manipulators. Mastery of two of the four techniques for each spinal region will enable the beginner to employ vertebral manipulation in his practice in safety, and with considerable expectation of success. He will make his own choice out of these to suit his particular needs, initially probably using only about half of them. He will modify them with experience; he may add more sophisticated techniques in time if he so wishes. Here, I am concerned with basic teaching only.

Their description is deliberately simple, without the use of specific jargon, so that orthodox physicians will understand clearly what is being attempted, and will not be discouraged by the use of terminology which smacks of the complementary. I am describing perfectly orthodox medical therapies in orthodox medical terms.

Some may be surprised that muscle energy techniques have not been included in this basic text. This is deliberate as they are not as easy to learn as the simple techniques described. Their exclusion from this text in no way implies that they are not useful in musculoskeletal practice, rather that they are better suited to subsequent courses.

Another cause for surprise may be that I advocate the teaching of thrust techniques for beginners. This again is deliberate, as I find these, on the whole, more effective than the non-thrust techniques, and the novice is thereby encouraged by his early successes. They are no more difficult to learn and they are not accompanied by added risks, so long as the contraindications to manipulation are at all times strictly observed.

Appendix 6
A choice of injections

Rationale for the inclusion of injections in this book

Injections were deliberately excluded from in-depth discussion in the workshop, as shortage of time demanded that we concentrated on manipulative techniques and their justification. However, they form an important part of the armamentarium of those concerned with musculoskeletal medicine. For this reason, I have included a selection of them in this appendix.

History

1. Local anaesthetics have been in use for more than 100 years.
2. It has been shown that their clinical effect commonly far exceeds their known pharmacological activity[72].
3. This is true in both degree and time.

Advantage to the medical profession

Injections are a form of therapy available to all doctors, and they are particularly appropriate to much of the work in general practice.

They are a simple quickly deployed first-line back-up to manipulation, currently NOT available to ancillary or complementary therapists. For this reason, they demand the serious consideration of all those involved with musculoskeletal medicine. In view of the widespread incidence of these very common problems, this means a high proportion of doctors.

Equipment

It is best to use the smallest syringe and the thinnest needle compatible with reaching the target. Not only is this kinder in terms of inflicting minimum additional pain but the use of large syringes and needles is terrifying to the patient and wholly unnecessary. And, of course, an anxious patient is not well relaxed, rendering any local therapy the more difficult.

Materials

This remains very much a matter of individual preference. There is little difference in effect between one local anaesthetic and another, between different strengths of solution, or between local anaesthetic alone, anaesthetic and steroid, normal saline and dry needling. Different steroids also make little difference to the outcome, which remains unpredictable!

Both inadvertent acupuncture and supratentorial factors are inevitably operative – the deeper the site, the more structures are stimulated en route; the bigger the needle, the more supratentorial stimulation is likely!

The relative proportions used in anaesthetic/steroid mixtures are of little importance, and there is no clear indication as to which mixture is best. There appears to be little advantage in long-acting steroids (if Mehta is right!)[73]. Recently, the Department of Health has raised a query as to the advisability of injecting steroids: this is yet to be resolved.

My personal preferences are:
Lignocaine (0.5%) + Cortistab for acute lesions
Lignocaine (0.5%) + triamcinolone for chronic lesions

Technique is extremely important. Apart from the desirability of a low concentration of both elements of the injection, the use of a test dose is a sensible safety precaution in case of unknown sensitivity to the drug. Pre-injection aspiration is vital in spinal injections, as this will reveal whether the needle has inadvertently punctured a blood vessel or even the theca. The lowest effective volume is advisable in all cases. In case of unexpected reactions, resuscitation facilities should be available at all times.

Peripheral nerve block

This is surprisingly seldom of great help in pain of vertebral origin, though perhaps of most use in rib fractures and persistent headaches. In the first case, wide infiltration into the periosteum adjacent to the fracture often proves more helpful than the nerve block itself. In the latter case, block of the greater occipital nerve of Arnold is almost incidental to wide local infiltration.

PRACTICAL – always inject widely around the intended spot – but is this nerve block at all? The most important factor here is that this does not matter!

Trigger points

These are a common phenomenon, although presenting under many guises (including non-existent fibrositis). There is no currently proven pathology, although they appear to be manifestations of referred tenderness, accompanied by local muscle spasm.

Much mystique has grown up around trigger points, at times proffered with great conviction. Travell has written extensively on the subject but firm evidence as to their nature is still to be found[74]. At least one clinician claims to move them about in a somewhat bizarre fashion by VERY forceful manipulation of the neck[75]!

Perhaps their most interesting feature is their close topographical correlation with acupuncture points for pain. This suggests a close association with the phenomenon of referred tenderness.

There is little point in detailing the common sites for their appearance, as, by their nature, these are very variable. However, they commonly respond to either manipulation or local injection. They should always be sought (see Chapter 11).

PRACTICAL – injection of trigger points is a simple therapy; injection should be made at the point of maximum tenderness! A vigorous rubbing of the area after the injection is often helpful.

Results of injection are commonly gratifying.

Attachment tissues

Injection of these is most valuable in practice, in particular occipital, scapular, brachial and spinal. This is in part because pain arising from attachment tissues is common. They are easy to confuse with trigger points as they may be situated in close proximity, and pressure sufficient to cause pain in one is enough to provoke the other: but does it matter? If the same treatment is to be applied, in the same place and with the same degree of unpredictability, the answer has to be NO.

Once more, the probing finger indicates the point for injection with unfailing accuracy, after being alerted by the history.

PRACTICAL – efficacy is usually immediately obvious to patient.

REMEMBER that the superficial part of the posterior ramus of L1 crosses the pelvic brim to innervate the upper buttock – it may become entrapped as it passes through the fascia[45]. While injection may often suffice, it occasionally warrants surgery. LOOK FOR LOCAL PHYSICAL SIGNS AT THE THORACO-LUMBAR JUNCTION. It may prove best to treat this region first.

REMEMBER that tenderness may be referred peripherally, for example to the lateral epicondyle of the humerus, secondary to pain of cervical vertebral origin. ALWAYS LOOK AT THE NECK FIRST, treating this first if local signs are present.

Posterior vertebral joints

Injection in the vicinity of the posterior vertebral joints may be extremely valuable in musculoskeletal medicine, particularly when manipulation is contraindicated. It is very easy to do at all levels from C2 downwards. I would never attempt C0/C1 or C1/C2.

Technique

It is easier to get angles right if the patient is prone.

The posterior joints are to be found about one (patient's) finger's breadth from the midline.

First, identify the point of maximum tenderness, marking the point with a ball-point pen or thumb nail; the latter is self-erasing!

In the neck, ensure that the cervical spine is in extension, in order to have the laminae overlapping, thus protecting against inadvertent epidural injection, or worse!

After an epidermal test dose, insert the needle at the point marked – VERTICALLY – press on until bone is reached – withdraw less than 1 mm before aspirating – in the absence of contraindications, inject half the dose – follow this by moving up to the posterior joint above, withdrawing partially only, leaving the needle still penetrating the skin, and repeat the process with one quarter of the dose, then repeat to the joint below, withdraw and rub the triple site vigorously. 1–2 ml is ample for this injection.

NOTE – There is no need to enter the joint; local diffusion will suffice – rub it! Neither is there any virtue in trying to enter the joint – nor much chance of your doing so!

The caudal epidural

This is by no means a new therapy. It was originally described in 1909!

Its object demands comment. Historically, it has been used diagnostically, on the assumption that the local anaesthetic molecule cannot penetrate the dura mater. This is unsound; in spite of this it continues to be taught that the dura is impermeable to the solutions injected, and that, therefore, if it works, the pain must have been of extradural origin (probably due to a disc protrusion)[76].

The truth about permeability of the dural sac is that it IS permeable, to the extent that the local anaesthetic molecule is present in the cerebrospinal fluid almost immediately, in the basal cisterns within minutes, and in the lateral ventricles within the hour, and that it penetrates the cord to at least 3 mm. It thus has NO diagnostic value. For further details, please see *Musculoskeletal Medicine, the Spine*[10].

Its only valid object in musculoskeletal medicine remains relief of pain of vertebral origin. The indication for its use is, therefore, severe lumbar and/or sciatic pain.

Its sole contraindication is sensitivity to local anaesthetics.

Its dangers, apart from sensitivity reactions and sepsis, are technical (e.g. entering a very abnormally long dural sac or damaging the cauda equina). Its complications are as for all injections.

As with other injections, the solution used is subject to both conflicting evidence and widely varying practice; it remains a very personal choice, guided largely by whim! However, in 1994, a warning was issued in the United Kingdom, which suggests that steroids may be detrimental[77]. It would be wise to omit them until the matter is clarified.

Technique

With the patient prone, first identify the posterior superior iliac spines, then identify the posterior inferior iliac spines and the sacral cornua. The sacral hiatus lies between the latter. Using a 21SWG needle, insert it in the midline over the hiatus, perpendicular to the skin surface, until the fibrous roof of the hiatus is felt to be just penetrated, then alter the angle of the needle to point rostrally, directly up the sacrum and insert the needle a further 2–3 cm. This angle will vary with the conformation of individual sacra.

Aspirate, alter the position of needle tip if necessary, and inject SLOWLY. If the patient reports pain on injection, give the remainder even MORE SLOWLY. Some clinicians like the patient to rest for variable periods after the injection, again governed largely by personal preference. It is certainly advisable that the patient does not drive a motor car for an hour or more.

Summary

Caudal epidural is a common useful office procedure, which may be repeated, if necessary, a number of times. However, if this seems to be becoming a habit, question whether it is the patient's habit or the clinician's! If the patient is 'hooked' on caudal epidurals, or if the clinician forgets how many he has done, it is time to think of something else! There is no point in continuing to give epidurals which are without long-term benefit to the patient.

There is no justification for regarding this simple technique as a minor surgical procedure.

Conclusion

Sclerosant injections have been excluded from this chapter as their indications rely upon somewhat dubious criteria. They are also unnecessarily painful for the patient. However, some clinicians hold them in high regard, and some patients seem to benefit from them.

On the other hand, local anaesthetic and 'mixed' injections are seen to be of substantial therapeutic potential, and, in particular, they offer the musculoskeletal physician a valuable option not currently available to lay manipulators. Further, they are all simple office procedures, requiring a minimum of equipment and time.

Appendix 7
Miscellaneous therapies available to the physician

Above all else, in the unpredictable event of vertebral manipulation not proving effective, the orthodox physician has at his disposal a great number of therapeutic options, apart from the variety of injections discussed in Appendix 6. In view of the fact that almost all therapy in the field of musculoskeletal medicine remains empirical, this must be of enormous advantage to the physician, and this advantage is reflected in his potential value to the patient. This is something which demands exploitation by the medical profession. No more than a brief outline of a selection of these therapies is given here to illustrate the breadth of choice enjoyed by the medical profession. A fuller selection of therapies is discussed in greater detail in *Musculoskeletal Medicine, the Spine*[10], where thirty therapies commonly of use in spinal pain are compared. Here, I refer only to those which are immediately applicable to general practice. Doctors wishing to take the matter further will find the appropriate references in the book quoted above.

The most readily prescribed are, of course, drugs. It is not necessary to do more than mention the four categories of drug which may play a part in the therapy of musculoskeletal disorders: the non-narcotic analgesics, the non-steroidal anti-inflammatory drugs, the psychotropic drugs (antidepressants, neuroleptics and tranquillizers) and the narcotics. Of course, all these groups are available (with certain restrictions) to the general practitioner, who is at once involved in the multiple problems of patient compliance, efficacy, undesirable side-effects, interaction between different drugs and cost.

Bedrest is very commonly prescribed, often unwisely! Its mode of operation in pain control is unknown and its value unpredictable, though it remains the only possible early treatment for some patients in the very acute stage of severe pain. It has, however, a number of potential dangers, particularly in the elderly, which need not be detailed here. Moreover, its use always disrupts the patient's life to a substantial degree, as it does that of his family and his livelihood. The optimum period of bedrest is as yet undetermined. It is therefore a therapy to be avoided if at all possible.

Collars and corsets are easily prescribed, again probably too often. There are certain reservations about how they work, it being clear that they do *not* prevent vertebral movement to a substantial degree, though they may act as a reminder not to move too much! Their variety is considerable, as is their cost. In the case of collars, there is the added danger of interference with the cervical reflexes, which may indirectly cause serious harm by loss of peripheral control in the dark or when driving motor cars. It is wise to prescribe them always with the intention of stopping their use at the earliest opportunity.

Various forms of physiotherapy are available, sometimes within general practice, sometimes only on referral to hospital or clinic. Direct referral to physiotherapists seems likely to increase in the United Kingdom, as a result of new directives from the Department of Health. But it should be remembered that none of these therapies are predictable in outcome, and that, arguably, the most likely to prove rapidly effective is vertebral manipulation, which the general practitioner may readily learn for himself.

Traction deserves a special mention, as it may well be available within general practice, and further it is perfectly feasible and frequently effective in DIY form, both for cervical and lumbar problems. DIY traction has the added advantages of requiring less of the doctor's therapeutic time, while involving the patient more with his own management (the latter a psychological bonus). A description of a simple apparatus is to be found in *An Introduction to Medical Manipulation*[78].

Acupuncture is a further therapy not to be dismissed, as it has its successes and is harmless. This applies also to electro-acupuncture and to transcutaneous electrical nerve stimulation. These three therapies (all of them involving A-fibre stimulation, with resultant C-fibre inhibition) lend themselves readily to general practice, and neither the capital cost nor the running costs of the necessary equipment is high.

Exercises are very widely employed in this field. No-one knows how they work! Without close supervision, what is practised may be far removed from what is prescribed! Over-zealous practice may cause harm; it is well to remember that irreparable damage may be caused to the intervertebral disc by the commonly used sit-up[18]. For this reason alone, it is probably wise to limit exercise to simple isometric routines, while stressing that they should be continued for life.

I have deliberately left hypnosis and relaxation routines to the end (and also the more complex psychotherapies) as they are all very time-consuming and therefore not entirely suited to general practice. Nonetheless, some doctors may find them very valuable, and they certainly have their places in the pain clinic.

It will be appreciated that, in spite of the frequent lack of diagnosis in this field resulting in his therapy being necessarily empirical, the doctor competent in manipulative and injection skills (apart from these additional ones) is in a particularly strong position to help his patient, by virtue of the variety of therapies at his disposal.

References

1. Campbell DG, Parsons CM. Referred head pain and its concomitants. J Nerv Ment Dis. 1944;99:544.
2. Jackson R. Headache associated with disorders of the cervical spine. Headache. 1967;6:175.
3. Prinzmetal M, Massumi RA. The anterior chest wall syndrome: chest pain resembling pain of cardiac origin. J Am Med Assoc. 1950;159:177.
4. Ashby EC. Abdominal pain of spinal origin. Ann RCS. 1977;59:242.
5. Paterson JK. Teaching within FIMM – the case for coordination. Presentation to the 11th International Congress of the Fédération Internationale de Médecine Manuelle, Bruxelles. 1992.
6. Paterson JK. An acceptable face to musculoskeletal medicine. Handbook for the first FIMM teachers' workshop, Vienna. 1994.
7. Paterson JK, Burn L, eds. Back pain, an international review. Lancaster: Kluwer Academic Publishers; 1990.
8. Davis C. Risks of manipulation. J R Soc Med. 1994;87(3):182.
9. Lewit K. Changes in locomotor function, complementary medicine and the general practitioner. J R Soc Med. 1994;87(1):36–9.
10. Burn L, Paterson JK. Musculoskeletal medicine: the spine. Lancaster: Kluwer Academic Publishers; 1990.
11. Paterson JK. "I can tell" – an impediment to progress in musculoskeletal medicine. J R Soc Med. 1994;87(11):648–9.
12. Wiltse LL. The effect of the common anomalies of the lumbar spine on disc degeneration and low back pain. Orthop Clin N Am. 1971;2:569–82.
13. Torgerson WR, Dotter WE. Comparative roentgenographic study of the asymptomatic and symptomatic lumbar spine. J Bone Jt Surg. 1976;58:850–3.
14. Collis JL, Ponseti IV. Long-term follow-up of patients with idiopathic scoliosis not treated surgically. J Bone Jt Surg. 1969;51:424–55.
15. Reading A. Testing pain mechanisms in persons in pain. In: Wall PD, Melzack R, eds. Textbook of pain. London: Churchill Livingstone; 1983.
16. Sternbach RA. Clinical aspects of pain. In: Sternbach RA, ed. Psychology of pain. New York: Raven Press; 1978.
17. Andersson S. In: Proceedings of the International Symposium organised by the National Back Pain Association. London. 1982.
18. Nachemson A. Lumbar intradiscal pressure. In: Jayson MIV, ed. The lumbar spine and low back pain. Tunbridge Wells, Pitman Medical; 1980.
19. Chaffin DB, Park KS. A longitudinal study of low back pain as associated with occupational weight lifting factors. Am Ind Hyd Assoc J. 1973;34:531–5.
20. Wilder DG, Woodworth BB, Frymoyer JW, Pope MH. Vibration and the human spine. Spine. 1982;7:243–54.
21. Wood PHN. The epidemiology of low back pain. In: Jayson MIV, ed. The lumbar spine and low back pain. Tunbridge Wells: Pitman Medical; 1980.
22. DuBoulay EPGH. Presentation to "The Bigots". 1989.
23. Nicholls PJR. Short leg syndrome. Br Med J. 1960:1:1863.
24. Paterson JK. The lateral index of sacral tilt. Presentations to the International Congresses of the Fédération Internationale de Médecine Manuelle. Prague/Zurich; 1982/3.
25. Kelsey JL. An epidemiological study of acute herniated lumbar discs. Rheumatol Rehabil. 1975;14:144–55.
26. Glover JR. Occupational health research and the problem of back pain. Occup Med. 1971;77:853.
27. Keele CA, Armstrong D. Substances producing pain and itch. London: Edward Arnold; 1964.
28. Lynn B. The detection of injury and tissue damage. In: Wall PD, Melzack R, eds. Textbook of pain. London: Churchill Livingstone; 1983.

29. Wall PD. The gate control theory of pain mechanisms: a re-examination of statements. Brain. 1978;101:1.
30. Wall PD. The laminar organisation of the dorsal horn and effects of descending impulses. J Physiol. 1967;188:403–23.
31. Carpenter. Differential supraspinal control of inhibitory and excitatory actions of the FRA to ascending spinal pathways. Acta Physiol Scand. 1965;63:103–10.
32. Bond MR. Psychology of pain. In: Andersson S et al., eds. Chronic non-cancer pain. Lancaster: MTP Press; 1987.
33. Kellgren JH. In: Copeman WSC, eds. Textbook of the rheumatic diseases, 5th edn. London: Pitman Medical; 1978.
34. Wyke B. The neurology of low back pain. In: Jayson MIV, ed. The lumbar spine and low back pain. Tunbridge Wells: Pitman Medical; 1980.
35. Denny-Brown D et al. The tract of Lissauer in relation to sensory transmission in the dorsal horn of the spinal cord in the macaque. J Comp Neurol. 1973;151:175.
36. Paterson JK, Burn L. Examination of the back, an introduction. Lancaster: MTP Press; 1986.
37. Wall PD. On the relation of injury to pain. Pain. 1979;6:253–64.
38. Leriche. The surgery of pain. Baltimore: Williams & Wilkins; 1939.
39. Bonica J. Important clinical aspects of acute and chronic pain. In: Beers, Bassett, eds. Mechanisms of pain and analgesic compounds. New York: Raven Press; 1979.
40. Craig. Emotional aspects of pain. In: Wall PD, Melzack R, eds. Textbook of pain. London: Churchill Livingstone; 1983.
41. Watson JP et al. Relationship between pain and schizophrenia. Br J Psychiatry. 1981;128:33–6.
42. McCreary C, Turner J, Dawson E. The MMPI as a predictor of response to conservative treatment for low back pain. J Clin Psychol. 1979;35:278–84.
43. Leavitt F, Garron DC. Validity of a back pain classification scale among patients with low back pain not associated with demonstrable organic disease. J Psychosom Res. 1979;23:301–6.
44. Graceley. Pain measurement in man. In: Bonica J, ed. Pain, common discomfort and humanitarian care. London: Elsevier; 1980.
45. Maigne J-Y. Entrapment of the cutaneous dorsal ramus of L1 or L2 and unilateral low back pain. An anatomical, clinical and surgical study. Prize presentation to the 11th International Congress of the Fédération Internationale de Médecine Manuelle, Bruxelles; 1992.
46. Porter RW et al. The shape and size of the lumbar canal. In: Proceedings of the Conference on Engineering Aspects of the Spine. London: Mechanical Engineering Publications; 1980.
47. Maigne R. Douleurs d'Origine vertebrale et traitements par manipulations. Paris: Expansion; 1992.
48. Fossgreen J. Presentation to symposium of the British Association of Manipulative Medicine, London; 1984.
49. Ashby EC. Abdominal pain of spinal origin. Ann R Coll Surg Eng. 1977;59:242.
50. Marinacci AA, Courville CB. Radicular syndromes simulating intra-abdominal surgical conditions. Am Surg. 1962;28:59.
51. LaRocca H, Macnab I. Value of pre-employment radiographic assessment of the lumbar spine. Can Med Assoc J. 1969;101:383.
52. Swezey RL, Silverman TR. Radiographic demonstration of induced vertebral facet displacement. Arch Med Rehabil. 1971;52:244.
53. Dove C. Presentation to the Colt Symposium, London; 1982.
54. Haldeman S. Presentation to the Colt Symposium, London; 1982.
55. White A, Panjabi M. Clinical biomechanics of the spine. Philadelphia: Lippincott; 1986.
56. Hilton RC. In: Jayson MIV, ed. The lumbar spine and low back pain, 2nd edn. Tunbridge Wells: Pitman Medical; 1980.
57. Moll J, Wright V. In: Jayson MIV, ed. The lumbar spine and low back pain, 2nd edn. Tunbridge Wells: Pitman Medical; 1980.
58. Keith A. Human embryology and morphology. London: Edward Arnold; 1948.
59. Basmajian JV, DeLuca CJ. Muscles alive. Baltimore: Williams & Wilkins; 1985.
60. Magora F, Magora A, Abramsky O, Goren B. An electromyographic investigation of the neck muscles in headache. Electromyogr Clin Neurophysiol. 1974;14:453–62.
61. Panjabi M. Presentation to the 8th International Congress of the Fédération Internationale de Médecine Manuelle, Madrid; 1986.

REFERENCES

62. Mixter WH, Barr JS. Rupture of intervertebral disc with involvement of the spinal cord. N Engl J Med. 1932;211:210.
63. Sylvest J, Hentzer B, Kobayasi T. Ultrastructure of prolapsed disc. Acta Orthop Scand. 1977;48:32–40.
64. Hitzelberger WE, Witten RM. Abnormal myelograms in asymptomatic patients. J Neurosurg. 1968;28:204.
65. Newman PH. The aetiology of spondylolisthesis. J Bone Jt Surg. 1963;45B:39.
66. Spangfort. In: Wall PD, Melzack R, eds. Textbook of pain. London: Churchill Livingstone; 1983.
67. Roaf R. Posture. London: Academic Press; 1978.
68. Janda V. Posture. Presentation to the FIMM Congress, Prague; 1982.
69. Andersson GBJ. Occupational aspects of low back pain. Presentation to the Colt Symposium, London; 1982.
70. Byrne JH. Mrs Byrne's dictionary of unusual, obscure and preposterous words. London: Granada Publishing; 1974.
71. Burn L. Manual of musculoskeletal medicine. Lancaster: Kluwer Academic Publishers; 1994.
72. Andersson S et al. Chronic non-cancer pain. Lancaster: MTP Press; 1987.
73. Swerdlow M, Mehta M. In: Anderson S, Bond M, Mehta M, Swerdlow M, eds. Chronic Non-Cancer Pain. Lancaster: MTP Press; 1987.
74. Travell J, Simons DC. Myofascial pain and dysfunction. The trigger point manual. Baltimore: Williams & Wilkins; 1983.
75. Fitzgerald RTD. Trigger Points. Presentation at the 10th FIMM Congress, Bruxelles; 1993.
76. Cyriax JH, Russell G. Textbook of orthopaedic medicine, 9th edn. London: Bailliere Tindall; 1977.
77. Government warning re injections. 1994.
78. Paterson JK, Burn L. An introduction to medical manipulation. Lancaster: MTP Press; 1985.

Index